The Old Man

and the **Road**

*Reflections While Completing
a Crossing of all 50 States
on Foot at Age 80*

by the author of ***Ten Million Steps***
and ***Go East Old Man***

Paul Reese

with Joe Henderson

Published by:
    Keokee Co. Publishing, Inc.
    P.O. Box 722
    Sandpoint, ID 83864
    Phone: 208/263-3573

Cover design by Deborah Vicari

Printed in the United States of America
10 9 8 7 6 5 4 3 2 1

Publisher's Cataloging-in-Publication Data
Reese, Paul, 1917-
    The old man and the road: reflections while completing a crossing of all 50 states on foot at age 80/by Paul Reese with Joe Henderson
    ISBN 1-879628-20-1
    1. Reese, Paul. 2. Running – United States – Biography. 3. Elderly – Physical Fitness – Biography. I. Henderson, Joe, 1943 – II. Title.
796.42' 092–dc20

Contents

To Elaine
for enough reasons to fill an encyclopedia

To Mark, Nancy and Susan
for encouragement and understanding

Prologue

An Overview

My affair with running across all 50 states might never have happened if, before I started, I had known the price — 7646 miles of running-jogging-walking, 558 days on the road (353 on foot), 60,000 miles of motorhome driving, considerable expense, and much exposure to danger and considerable inconvenience and discomfort.

Lucky that before starting I was not aware of the price and thus it was not a deterrent. As a result my wife Elaine and I (she driving a motorhome and pit-crewing for me, and I running) injected major adventure into our lives while crossing each of the 50 states.

Actually for us running across all 50 states was not the result of any Grand Scheme or Master Plan. Instead it evolved by bits and pieces in three distinct phases.

Phase One was a 3192-mile run across the USA in 1990 at age 73. On this run I was obsessed with getting from the Pacific Ocean (at Jenner, California) to the Atlantic Ocean (at Hilton Head Island, South Carolina). I gave no thought to running across states per se, although I did cross 12. Joe Henderson and I described this experience in our book *Ten Million Steps*.

Phase Two focused on running across the 14 states in the Lower 48 west of the Mississippi (Alaska and Hawaii were not in this equation) that I hadn't crossed on the USA run. In this case crossing a state meant crossing the full width of it, north to south or east to west, whichever was the shorter. These runs, done in summers (1992-96) were between the ages of 75 and 79. In our book *Go East Old Man* we described these adventures.

Phase Three, done at age 80, targeted completing running across the remaining 21 states east of the Mississippi I had not crossed previously, plus Alaska and Hawaii. These states are the focus of this final book in the trilogy, *The Old Man and the Road*. (At the end of the book I also review the five states east of the Mississippi that I crossed in earlier runs.)

With age catching up with me and with energy ebbing after my 80th birthday, I spent considerable time and energy seeking the shortest route across each of the final 23 states. However, I did adhere to the criterion that the run be across the state from the boundary of one state to the boundary of another state.

The route could be north-south or east-west. And a water boundary (such as the Atlantic Ocean for the east boundary of New Jersey or Lake Erie as the north boundary of Ohio) could be used. The point – and I don't want to fly under false colors here – is that I took the shortest route I could find.

My only regret here is that in two or three instances this route did not go across the state north-south or east-west but cut the state on a diagonal while starting at one state boundary and finishing at another. Frankly the main reason I took the shortest route was I felt that time was running out on me and I wanted to ensure reaching our goal of running across all 50 states. I finished the odyssey in December 1997.

A surprising number of athletes have run a marathon in each of the 50 states (that would equate to approximately 1311 miles) and another surprising number have run across the country. But to my knowledge I am the only person to have run across all 50 states.

For certain I am the *oldest* person to do that, as well as to have run across the USA. Those are my distinctions (just doing it, and age) because fast I was not, nor did I record any day longer than 32 miles. Hundreds of runners could do it better (meaning faster and taking longer routes). I'm just the old guy who ran across each of the states.

Not a day goes by without Elaine and me thanking God that we were able to do it and, while in slow motion, to see, to enjoy, to appreciate and come to more understand this great country of ours. Elaine and I sure as hell have been lucky. So much so that we should thank God twice a day, or more.

Speaking of thanks, I owe a heap. First to Joe Henderson who, in editing our three books, gave unduly of his time, expertise and patience. I admire him greatly as an editor but cherish him even more as a friend.

I also owe a vote of thanks to Chris Bessler and the staff of Keokee Publishing Company. Working with them has been a very pleasant experience.

And, going back in time, I say thank you to Dr. Wayman Spence of the WRS Group because when he was in the business of publishing inspirational books, he launched our trilogy with *Ten Million Steps*. For certain our three books would never have been published without the help of Joe, Chris, Billie Jean, Deborah and Wayman. Bless 'em all!

Paul Reese
Auburn, California
July 1999

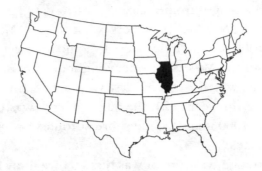

Illinois

*From the Mississippi River
to the Ohio River*

Dates: *April 28th to 30th, 1997*
Miles: *57.1*
Route: *Start on east bank of Mississippi River, go east on Ware/Wolf Road to Highway 146, then follow 146 to Golconda and Ohio River.*

DAY ONE.

> *At 40 I lost my illusions,*
> *At 50 I lost my hair,*
> *At 60 my hope and teeth were gone,*
> *And my feet were beyond repair,*
> *At 80 life has clipped my claws,*
> *I'm bent and bowed and cracked,*
> *But I can't give up the ghost because*
> *My follies are intact.*

Those words of E. Y. Harburg brought on smiles as Elaine and I, accompanied by our two Labradors, Rebel and Brudder, left home three days after my 80th birthday and headed for the eastern USA where my agenda called for running across the remaining 21 states east of the Mississippi. Were we setting out foolishly or valiantly, I kept asking myself?

I garnered strength from realizing that to date I'd run across 27 states (12 on RUNXUSA, 14 others west of the Mississippi, and Florida) for a total of 6812 miles. Here I should interject that there are 26 states east of the Mississippi, including four I crossed on the USA run and Florida, which I crossed last October – thus bringing the number to cross this year to 21. The question now was, could I handle another 800 to 1000 miles (taking shortest routes I could find) to get across these states?

The only thing I was sure of was that I'd give it my best. Come to think of it, there was a second thing Elaine and I were sure of: We had no desire to drive the motorhome all the way to the East Coast once again after this trip.

After communicating with people on the scene of many of our state routes and after much map study, Elaine and I had plotted a route across each state and then worked out our routing for getting from state to state. Seeing how the miles stacked up, we realized the motorhome would be every bit as tired as we.

The immediate task at hand as we left home was to drive 2200 miles to Illinois, where we'd launch our expedition. Both Elaine and I were anxious to get the show on the road because therein, as apart from simply driving across the country, lies the adventure and excitement.

Arriving in Illinois after seven days of motorhome travel from California, I was more than ready to start running. Time and again, I kept thinking, I've got 21 eastern states to run this spring and summer. Time to get the show on the road.

Back in the planning stage for this year's runs I had studied Illinois for a route and immediately noticed that the shortest would be in the southern portion of the state where it is the narrowest. The longest (390 miles) and widest (210 miles) parts of the state were to be avoided like the plague. Another thing for sure, I did not have to worry about big hills – the highest point in the state is 1,235 feet.

As I studied southern Illinois, Highway 146 loomed as one of the shortest routes across the state. Next question: Was it runnable?

To find out, I asked John McKeown, a Marine Corps classmate with whom I had gone through officer training. John and his wife Doakie, an upbeat and outgoing couple, live in Decatur, Illinois, and are familiar with the state.

John wrote, "Yes, Route 146 should be a decent run across Illinois.

It's beautiful country – rolling hills, partly wooded, much of the land is federal parkland.

"Before you arrive, better practice pronouncing Vienna. Like this: *Vie-enna* (long 'i') – who knows why? Watch the park benches in Vienna as you pass – you'll see pictures of retired Senator Paul Simon. It's his home."

John's analysis of Highway 146 was reinforced by Bill Short, Jr., District Operations Engineer for the Illinois Department of Transportation, who told me, "Most of the shoulders on Illinois 146 are dirt or sod. The western part of Illinois Route 146 (west of Interstate 57) is fairly heavily traveled, but traffic falls off as you proceed east.

"There are no large city complexes. The largest city is Anna with a population of 5000. Illinois 146 east of Anna is comprised at times of very hilly terrain with narrow shoulders."

Southern Illinois is bracketed by the Mississippi River on the west and the Ohio River on the east. My run would be from river to river.

On the west side I had two choices of where to start: I could start at Cape Girardeau (oh boy, a chance to see the boyhood home of Rush Limbaugh!), or I could start on the banks of the Mississippi near the hamlet of Ware. Easy decision because the Ware start was roughly 10 miles shorter – no offense to Rush here.

As for Cape Girardeau, a native of the city told me that the bridge over the Mississippi there has been toll-free since 1956. As we drove over it on our way to Ware, it appeared to date back to the days of Abe Lincoln.

To get to the banks of the Mississippi from Ware, I had to leave Highway 146 at Ware and go a little more than three miles westward on a paved, then gravel and dirt roads. As I stood on the river bank and looked at the formidable body of water, I was glad I was not a pioneer who had to devise a way to cross this intimidating barrier.

I had no trouble suppressing an urge to swim to the middle of the river which would be exact boundary between states. I wished Elaine were beside me to share the view, but she was half a mile away because the dirt road to the bank did not appear receptive to the motorhome.

Getting underway, I found myself entertaining two dominant thoughts. First, joyful that the planning and anticipating were over and that we were now launching our 21-state expedition. Second, some concern over whether I would hold up to cover (by running, jogging, walking – in descending order of desirability – whichever I could muster) these remaining states east of the Mississippi. I readily and reluctantly recognized that between the ravages of aging and asthma, my stamina arsenal was dwindling.

In our planning Elaine and I had calculated that our route across Illinois would be somewhere between 57 and 60 miles. Which lead to the decision to break this distance into three days of running. Probably as a result of my adrenaline pumping from the excitement of starting our summer safari, I was a tad overambitious our first day by logging 22.3 miles.

The dominant thought that I took away from the day's run was that most Americans think of Illinois in stereotypes – Chicago, Lake Michigan, O'Hare (the world's busiest airport), Sears Tower (the world's tallest building) – and, oh yes, the Chicago Bulls. The flip side of this thinking is that most of Illinois is given over to agriculture. The state ranks first in the production of soy beans and second to Iowa in corn production.

Other agriculture products, many of which I saw today, include barley, wheat, oats, asparagus, onions, tomatoes, berries, peaches and apples. As further evidence of the local agriculture a number of fruit stands were spaced along my route today.

I noticed that all the farms were neatly kept, and I got the impression they were all small holdings. Nothing resembled the extensive agriculture holdings seen in such states as Montana, Wyoming and Nebraska.

There was a touch of diversion from agriculture along the way when I passed through Jonesboro and Anna, two adjacent cities. Anna, with 5000 citizens, is almost three times bigger than Jonesboro and certainly the livelier of the two. Jonesboro's claim to fame, a historical marker told me, lies in its being the scene of one of the Lincoln-Douglas debates.

To me the most distinctive feature of Anna was a number of stately homes. Some of those on the east side of town could be called small mansions. It would be hard even on driving fast through Anna, as apart from running, not to notice that the city is studded with churches of all denominations.

On the road my curiosity was whetted when I saw historical markers referring to the Trail of Tears. Checking this out, I found the reference was to the 1838 winter death march of the Cherokee nation. Five thousand people died on the journey when President Andrew Jackson ordered the Cherokees removed from the fertile Tennessee Valley to the arid plains of Oklahoma.

On much of the road today with its dips, curves and only tall grass for a shoulder, the running conditions were not joyful. But the scenery, while not spectacular, remained pleasant all day. Being in this serene setting – removed from the hurly-burly of cities and the roar of freeway traffic – was peaceful.

Jogging along, engrossed with the setting, thinking about the states that lay ahead, grooving into the pit-crew routine with Elaine, I moved through the day without feeling undue strain or pain. It was only after I finished and while we were driving to the state park to overnight that I realized I was tired from overrunning today. It was a delightful feeling, though, to have weathered the first day with all body components uncomplaining, albeit a bit tired – and beyond that to have finally started something we'd been thinking about for months.

It could even be said that I was living the Bible because, to quote Ecclesiastes, "Every man should... enjoy the good of his labor; it is the gift of God."

I went to bed doing just that. Even more, I went to sleep feeling good about this day.

DAY TWO. When I was about to start today, I found myself thinking it was somewhat appropriate that, being tired yesterday, I finished relatively close to a cemetery, one about which I made three observations: The name, McGinnis Cemetery struck me as odd; the headstones were of a rich marble, and most of the graves were decorated with artificial flowers, a custom which until now I had thought prevailed in the South.

I had not gone very far this second day when I felt something stepping on one of my heels. Turning around, I saw two dogs, a Doberman and a German Shepherd both – and sing hallelujah here – in a playful mood! I gave them some of the attention they were seeking, then, hoping to remove them from the danger of the highway, told them, "Go home!" Tremendous command presence because they obeyed instantly.

For some reason, this dog commentary reminded me of remarks made by Jeremiah Russell while roasting me at my 80th birthday party on April 17th. Jeremiah, a running friend and retired high school English teacher, scorched me by joking about how *Ten Million Steps*, the book on my USA run, was heavy with commentary about road kill, snakes and the foul smell of rendering plants.

I didn't get a chance to rebut Jeremiah, but if I had I might have said: My snake phobia is traceable to my grandmother who, while fetching water at a creek on the ranch, saw a rattlesnake, fainted, and drowned. Road kill is a constant reminder of my own affinity with death while on the road. The foul smell of a rendering plant gets to me because, endowed with a prominent proboscis, I'm super sensitive to such smells.

However, since Elaine is already planning my 90th birthday party (yep, she does believe in projecting!) and since Jeremiah will most likely be there again to roast me, out of deference to him (no guarantees here!) I have resolved to refrain from snake/roadkill/rendering plant commentary as I trudge through Illinois.

The dogs also reminded me of another animal observation. When I went past Pride Acres, I saw 15 horses grazing on the grassy slopes, and the sight was so striking that even Dick Francis would stop to take a second look at this thoroughbred horseflesh.

Around four miles this second day I was surprised to come upon a stretch of road where the area resembled a Louisiana bayou. Just flooded lowlands with lots of trees, I decided. Nevertheless, I kept a sharp lookout for alligators (ye gods, now at my 90th party Jeremiah will accuse me of harping on alligators!).

Road and running conditions today were about the same as those that characterized yesterday – two-lane road, fog line exactly at the edge of the road and beyond it tall grass on the shoulder, a dipsy-doodle road with many ups and downs. A compensating factor was that all the drivers moved over for me.

Well, let me amend that: All the drivers west of Vienna moved over, but in the short span between Vienna and I-24 to the east, none moved over. I puzzled over the sociological significance of that.

Speaking of Vienna, I actually detoured a half-mile out of my way to wander into the town's business district in order to look for the Paul Simon benches that John McKeown had mentioned to me. Not one such bench did I see.

To prove I was on the scene, I did stop to take a picture of the Johnson County Courthouse, a brick building as ancient as I. Also, John in mind, I asked a native how the town's name was pronounced and confirmed it was precisely as he had stated, long "i" in the Vienna.

Elaine and I had no awareness until we stumbled onto them that the Shawnee Correctional Facility (medium security) and Vienna Correctional Facility (minimum security) were located on our route. Elaine, parked near Shawnee for a pit stop, got firsthand awareness when one of the guards drove out to check on her.

As the day went on, I discovered that one hazard of the route was ticks. Each time after I stepped out on the grass to avoid an oncoming car, I checked my legs for ticks and in the course of the day peeled off close to a dozen.

Thoughts of Arnold Schwartzenegger and his recent heart operation drifted into my head today as I wandered down the road. This would have been an absolute shocker had it not been for the similar experience of Ralph Paffenbarger, an MD friend of mine.

After so many experiences of running with Paff in the hills, where the man was a virtual animal, I could hardly believe it when he was felled with a faulty heart valve that had to operated on. Paff's experience made Arnold's easier for me to understand.

Speaking of Arnold, he's thought of in stereotype by the American public as Mr. Macho instead of as the highly intelligent, sophisticated, caring, gentleman par excellence that he is. At least that is my observation of him when I, as a consultant, attend the meetings of the California Governor's Council on Physical Fitness and Sports which he chairs.

We finished our 19.3-mile day in Grantsburg, a hamlet which harbored only a post office and Jim's Trading Post. Seeking entertainment, and responding to Elaine's "dare you," I ventured into Jim's and saw an inventory of clothing, shoes, notions, books, records and hardware that had been on hand long enough, I guessed, to have grown fungus.

A musty smell permeated the poorly lit room. Though I stayed but a brief time, I felt upon leaving that I was a candidate for fumigation.

From Grantsburg, we had another 25 or so miles of driving to get to Dixon Springs State Park to roost for the night. The park had 80 RV spaces, and we were the only customers – proving April is a great time of year to travel.

DAY THREE. We were awakened early the next morning by a chorus of chanting. Investigating, we found that the Dixon Springs Correctional Facility was next door and that it has a program with some aspects of boot camp where the prisoners run and chant. The ones we saw, all wearing red jumpsuits, were moving at a good clip.

When I departed Grantsburg about 8:30 A.M., I took some satisfaction from knowing that by the end of this day, one that turned out to be 15.5 miles, we would have completed one of the 21 eastern states on our docket.

Often during the day I dwelt on how peaceful it was on this road far removed from the hurly-burly of a big city, from the roar of traffic on an Interstate. Crossing the state, I must have waved an acknowledgment to at least 200 drivers who moved over for me and each in return waved back. Will Rogers said, "I never met a person I didn't like." Ditto for me and Illinois drivers – except for those zombies between Vienna and I-24.

Elaine never ceases to surprise me. Today as I passed a chocolate factory (the woman is a chocolate addict), she was not parked there stocking up on candy. Utterly unpredictable!

My Boy Scout deed of the day was taking a turtle, about four inches in diameter from the middle of the road where he was automobile fodder, and carrying him safely to the other side of the road. Doing so, I noticed that he had a colorful shell and, thankfully, excellent bladder control!

Again today I could not help but notice that the lowlands along this route are filled with water and resemble a bayou. I suspect this is year-round and not just flooding.

I had a short dialogue with a farmer today who saw my T-shirt reading "Running Across All 50 States". The conversation went like this:

He: "Does that shirt mean what it says?"

Me: "Yes, but at this point jogging would be more appropriate than running."

He:"Why in the world would you do a thing like that. It seems like a waste of time. Especially at your age."

Me:"I guess the main reason I do it is because I enjoy it."

He:"Well, to each his own. It just seems like a waste of valuable time to me."

And with that he climbed back onto his nearby tractor and drove off. Ah yes, nothing like a bit of encouragement!

In the 28 states I've run across to date, I've never seen mileage marked as precisely as in Illinois. Fact is, it took me a while to become aware of the mileage signs and to decipher them (okay, so I'm a slow learner). The signs, all recorded by county, consist of a circle across the center of which is the name of the county, above that the name of the highway and below the county name the mileage.

For example, the road I'm on would read at the top 146, middle Union County, bottom 19.00 meaning 19 miles. One of these signs appears at every crossroad, such as 19.52.

Nearing the finish at Golconda, I was not sure of the shortest way to get to the Ohio River, our finish spot. So I stopped to inquire at a convenience store on the west edge of town.

"Very easy," Bob Dover told me. "Just straight ahead for 1000 yards and you're at the river."

Seeing my T-shirt , he wanted to know if I was running for a cause or sponsor. He found it hard to believe that I was doing it for sheer enjoyment.

Going through town on the way to the river, I made note of the Rottman Funeral Home. Reflecting on it, I thought maybe a name change here would be appropriate.

The town, called Quilt City (little wonder since quilts were for sale in every store), appeared battered and old. I saw a pharmacy, no grocery store, and a number of empty store fronts.

I was not prepared for what I saw when I came to the river levee, this being the east border of Golconda and Illinois. I was stupefied at the size of the Ohio River. An awesome sight.

The Ohio, I realized, must have been a boon to early settlers in being a navigable freeway for transportation. And yet, being so formidable, it was a monstrous impediment to movement westward.

Later when I visited the Pope County building in town, I told Evelyn Hogg, county clerk and recorder, that the water seemed unusually high. "You should have seen it two weeks ago," she replied. "Almost to the top of the levee."

She added that back in 1913 and again in 1937 the river did flood. The '37 flood did severe damage to Golconda.

She also told me that the town dated back to 1797 when Major James Lusk operated a ferry here across the Ohio River. The town was originally named Sarahville after Lusk's widow, In 1817 the County Court ordered that the name change to Golconda.

Looking back on Illinois, it is as best I can remember, the first state I've run across without finding any money whatsoever and without having any police officer (state, county, or city) stop to check on either Elaine or me.

All told, despite the less than desirable road shoulders, it was a comfortable run. The state parks, all excellent facilities, were spaced so that we averaged only around 25 miles on our drives to the start and from the finish.

And the natives were friendly. A nice baptism for the 20 eastern states to follow!

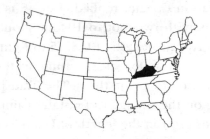

Chapter 2

Kentucky

My Kentucky Derby

Dates: *May 1st to 3rd, 1997*
Miles: *47.6*
Route: *Start at Tennessee/Kentucky border on Highway 97 and follow 97 north to Mayfield and Highway 121. North on 121 to Highway 45, then follow 45 to Paducah and Ohio River, north Kentucky border.*

DAY ONE. My earliest memories of Kentucky go back to my grammar school days when I was trying dutifully but dismally to learn to play the piano. "My Old Kentucky Home" was a song I slaughtered with regularity while practicing. In subsequent years I learned that Kentucky is noted for its horses, bluegrass, Kentucky Derby, bourbon and tobacco.

In other words, when I set about to plan a running route across Kentucky, I knew very little about the state. In fact, my knowledge of the state ranked on par with my rendition of "My Old Kentucky Home."

It didn't take long for me to recognize, after studying a map of Kentucky, that one of the shortest running routes across the state would be one that started on Highway 97 at the Tennessee border and went north to Highway 45 and into Paducah, thence to the Illinois border at the Ohio River. This route in mind, I contacted the Transportation Cabinet (called the Department of Transportation in most states) and also a runner living in the state for info about the route. The answers I received from both left questions in my mind.

The Transportation Cabinet replied, "U.S. 45 is a combination of two and four lanes with two-foot to 10-foot shoulders." A permit is required to legally run the length of U.S. 45 in Kentucky.

"We have had requests for such permits in the past, and it has been our practice not to grant them. The Transportation Cabinet considers running on the shoulder of a state maintained route to be unsafe. If you choose to run the length of U.S. 45 in Kentucky, it will be without a legal permit."

The runner replied, "Highway 45 looks very feasible to me. Mayfield, Kentucky, is a pretty rough town, but I really don't think you will have any problems. As statistics point out, homicides or assaults are perpetrated by local family members against each other, rarely is a stranger assaulted."

"Have a good run and try to pick a day that rain is not forecast. There are no mountains in that area, and it's tornado country."

Decision time: Should I chance getting cited by the Kentucky Highway Patrol and flirting with a confrontation in Mayfield? The alternative would be to seek another route, one that would add at least 50 miles more. The shortest distance (around 48 miles) on 97/45 was a reality, whereas citing and confrontation were only possibilities. I decided to take a chance on 97/45.

Accordingly on May 1st, the day after finishing Illinois, I found myself in Kentucky on Highway 97 at the Tennessee border and headed north toward Paducah. As I took my first steps, the words "Carry me back to good old Paducah not so far away" came to mind.

Try as I might, I could not recall the song that contained these lines. Too bad, I thought, that my longtime friend, Bill Glackin, was not nearby. Bill's been a critic for the *Sacramento Bee* for more than 40 years, and he could name the song instantly.

I had gone less than a mile when a lady walking toward me cautioned, "Watch our for poisonous snakes. These are the bottoms, you know."

By the "bottoms" I guessed she was referring to the delta basin. No, Lady, I didn't know. If I had, I might be elsewhere.

Damn it, the lady is right, I thought at two miles when I came across a four-foot snake sunning itself in the middle of the road. As if that were not enough, I got another dose of snake when I talked with J.E. Foy who warned me, "Be careful out here. Copperheads and water moccasins are abundant down in the bottoms."

He was a gentleman I'd guess to be in his early 60s, quite dapper in jeans and a plaid shirt, who told me he'd spent his entire life within a 15-mile radius of our meeting spot on the road. "The average farm around here," he informed me in answer to my question, "is 50 to 60 acres. No more."

The battle plan today was to cover the 17-mile stretch from Highway 97 and the Tennessee border to Mayfield. This would leave us around 30 miles to do on Highways 121 and 45, the Kentucky Highway Patrol permitting.

The only person I talked with other than J.E. Foy was a young farmer, who looked to be in his mid-20s. He stopped and yelled to me, "Looks like you're going a long ways."

"Oh, not too far," I replied.

"Where you going to?"

"To the Illinois border."

"How far is that?"

"I'd guess around 40 miles."

"Boy, that's a long ways", he said as he drove off. As he left, I thought it somewhat strange that I should be telling a native how far it is to the nearby Illinois border.

While parked for pit stops today, Elaine had conversations with two people – a farmer and a high school girl. Elaine was parked beside a fence admiring the cows nearby when a farmer approached her and learned what she was doing.

"You want to see them closer?" he asked. Then without waiting for an answer, he yelled, "C'mon, c'mon." On that command all the cows ambled to the fence where Elaine was.

At the 16-mile mark a high school girl came out of her home to talk with Elaine who was parked waiting for me. They had a long conversation in which Elaine told her about my running.

Elaine must have given me quite a buildup because the girl said, "I want his autograph just in case he becomes famous someday."

Elaine enjoyed the visit so much that she decided to go one step further and give her a copy of our book, *Ten Million Steps*, autographed by me. I inscribed, "Best wishes, Becky, and onward to college." I made the college reference because Elaine told me that the girl planned to attend Murray State College nearby.

"The highlight of my day," Elaine reported, "was watching that girl's eyes light up when I handed her the book."

For all intents and purposes, I was in an agricultural setting all day. Immediately after getting started, I passed a number of extremely modest homes near the levee road – at $20,000 they would have been overpriced – all of which had considerable junk strewn around their yards. But by the time I reached two miles, there was a transition to nice middle-class homes, all well kept.

The Kentucky map had told me that I'd pass through Bell City, Tri City and Sedalia, and I had hoped to see some interesting sights. Not so, though.

All I saw in Bell City was the Church of Christ, the Bell City Pottery Works and Bell City Baptist Church – the last a brick building and nicest structure seen in these parts.

Tri City was a puzzler because all I saw here, at the junction of Highways 97/94, was a gas station and a convenience store. No city. I reasoned that the name Tri City came from this being a crossroads to three cities: Fulton 24 miles west, Murray 12 miles east, and Mayfield 14 miles north.

Sedalia consisted of three churches, Bob and Ann's Grocery, a post office, elementary school and Sedalia Restaurant. Period.

I asked a native, "Where do the kids here go to high school?"

His answer, "In Mayfield. It's seven miles from here."

A bit of diversion from the road routine was introduced when I saw a basalite building that at first glance I judged to be a fruit stand. As I got closer, I read the sign on it: "STOP. SEE A ROAD MAP TO HEAVEN."

Then, looking into the building, I saw another sign behind the picnic table in the patio area. This sign read, "Road map to heaven. What must I do to be saved?"

Then followed a list of six steps, the full biblical text written on a marble plaque. Summarized (for those wanting to take the trip!) they were:

1. Hear the gospel (Paul)
2. Believe in the gospel (Paul)
3. Repent (Luke)
4. Confess Christ (Matthew)
5. Be baptized (no source given)
6. Continue faithful unto death (no source)

Felt sort of lucky today after realizing that Elaine had passed by the Pleasant Hills Kennels, breeders of Labradors, and had not stopped to pick up a yellow Lab to go with her brown and black Labs.

Being aware that Kentucky is known for its horses and also aware that, dating from the days of Adolph Rupp, Kentucky is known for its basketball teams, I took note of two oddities today: I saw not one horse, nor one basketball hoop.

The first dozen miles today were relatively easy, but the last five were difficult because traffic increased considerably. More often than desired, I had to stand in the tall grass, exposed to ticks and snakes, waiting for cars to pass.

After finishing this first day, we had no choice but to drive 30 miles to Ken Lake State Park in Aurora, Kentucky, the nearest facility for RV camping. We were shown that the Kentucky state parks are top drawer.

DAY TWO. Our second day in Kentucky, another 17-mile effort, brought us to within 13.6 miles of Paducah and the Illinois border. I had two problems this day. One was anxiety over whether the Kentucky Highway Patrol would cite me for running on Highway 45, and the other was running most of the day in a heavy rainstorm.

I felt lucky, though, just to be on the road after the asthma attack that hit me around three A.M. During the entire episode, lasting an hour or so, I was gasping for breath, not sure I'd get my next one, hacking, coughing, trying to expel phlegm.

Using inhalants and coffee as my weapons, I tried to counter-attack. Watching me under siege, Elaine was not too sure that I would survive.

Now fast forward four hours or so, and here I was on the road jogging. Almost miraculous.

When I tell an MD about the ferocity of one of these attacks and that Elaine, watching, considers me on the verge of death, he looks at me incredulously and his unspoken words are, "Oh, c'mon, it can't be that bad or you wouldn't be able to do the running you do." I'm sure that many of the asthmatic Olympians who have won medals have gone through the same routine.

The most variety of the day occurred along Highway 121, the connecting link between Highways 97 and 45, which routes through

Mayfield. The southern end of 121 was lined with fast food joints, the most unusual of which was the Sonic Drive-in.

This is a throwback to the drive-ins of the 1950 where each customer parks by his individual microphone and orders. Popular as Sonics seem to be east of the Mississippi, I don't recall ever seeing one west of it.

Going through downtown Mayfield, 121 was a traffic nightmare as it circled the town square housing the county courthouse, post office and other public buildings. I ran past traffic bottlenecked for five blocks.

In Mayfield I saw nothing distinctive or impressive, nor did I see any evidence of it being "a rough town" about which I had been fore-warned. I did, though, see some very elaborate homes on Highway 121 shortly after leaving the town square.

A mile or so from downtown, Highway 121 connected with Highway 45, and as I trudged up the ramp to 45 I was hopeful that the Highway Patrol would ignore my presence. Immediately I was taken with how safe 45 was, a divided road with two lanes on each side and breakdown lane, which is about as safe as running on a highway can get.

Surprisingly during my entire time on 45 this day I did not see a Kentucky Highway Patrol officer driving in either direction. The fates are indeed kind!

As for the rain it provided one amusing incident. At one point, to escape a torrential downpour and to take refuge from the lightning and thunder, I took shelter under an overpass. I was there a few minutes when I saw that about eight feet away I had a companion, a four-foot snake trying to keep dry. Applauding my bravery at tolerat-ing this proximity, I kept an eye on him and relaxed only after he departed.

Running on Highway 45 today was somewhat humdrum – but safe. Also a bit sterile since I had no contacts with people and was removed from places.

Along the way I did take note of a huge General Tire Plant, a key contributor to Mayfield's economy, of the Mid-continent Baptist College and its sprawling brick structures, and of Seaboards, a huge agricultural processing plant.

By the time we reached 17 miles, the rain, thunder and lightning were so threatening that we decided to quit for the day and drive into Paducah and scout for a route that would take us directly to the river and the Illinois border. That done, we overnighted at Fern Lake RV Park, near Paducah.

DAY THREE. Nice feeling, my third day in Kentucky, to know that I had only 13.6 miles left to finish the state. Had to admit that on this mileage I felt a bit wimpish. In years previous to this I would have finished Kentucky in two days rather than three.

Somewhat of a good feeling this morning – after last night's torrential rain, flood warning and tornado alert – just to be on the road unscathed, even though the wind and temperature in the high 30s chilled me.

Now that we're into our sixth day of running (three in Illinois, three in Kentucky), I've noticed a new pattern developing, one that reflects Elaine's philosophy, "This is a vacation." The pattern is that nowadays we begin our runs around 8:00 or 8:30 in the morning.

Quite a contrast to our RUNXUSA days when I was on the road around five o'clock running by flashlight. From USA we moved to the "states west of the Mississippi expedition" during which we were on the road at seven A.M. Lucky we don't have another summer of this, or we'd probably hit the road after lunch!

An early thought on the road today went back to 33 years ago when I ran my first long-distance race. When I came around the first corner, a young runner yelled to me, "Be careful, old man, or you'll kill yourself at that pace."

Ye gods, I was a mere child of 47 at the time. Now that I'm 80 and running across states, I wonder what that guy would say.

Ah yes, that first race, I remember it well: 15 miles, temperature 88 degrees, and not a single aid station on the entire course. I was weaned tough to distance running!

I saw him only after he passed by me, a Kentucky state trooper in a gray vehicle, and blessings on him for not stopping. Could it be that he was hurrying to the Kentucky Derby, which is today? By far the most enjoyable sight of the day for me was watching him speed away.

Several times this day I reflected on how comfortable and safe I felt running on a divided highway while protected by a breakdown lane. Ironically highway and transportation departments harbor the erroneous belief that a runner is safer on a less traveled two-lane road, though it has no shoulder and the runner is prey to getting hit by a car passing from behind him.

It seemed that everywhere I looked on Highway 45 I saw greenery – the grass in the median, the forestation on both sides of the road and some glimpses of agriculture as it appeared through openings in the forestation.

I was rudely jolted from this serenity when I came into the Paducah environs. In one area, because the traffic was so heavy and the road offered no running space, I resorted to running three blocks through a cemetery and in doing so I discovered that Alben Barkley, vice-president and Senate majority leader under Franklin Roosevelt and vice-president under Harry Truman, is buried there.

A plaque told me he died April 30th, 1956, while addressing a mock Democratic convention at Washington and Lee University. His last words were, "I'd rather be a servant in the house of the Lord than sit in the seats of the mighty."

Leaving the cemetery, I was forced to run on the grassy yards of homes because the road was without a bike lane and none of the approaching drivers would move over for me, despite the fast lane being empty. I suspected their failure was not due to being impolite or uncaring but instead simply because they were not thinking. This long stretch of city space with no sidewalks, no place for pedestrians, I labeled as a testimonial to the American fixation with motorization and lack of regard for providing paths for exercise.

After a mile or so of running through the cemetery and residential yards, I came to sidewalks that provided running space all the way to the river and the border. I had to be careful not to trip because the sidewalks were in dire need of repair.

One impression I got while heading toward downtown was that there seems to be overkill with hospital facilities in Paducah. When I first saw the Lourdes Hospital, eight stories or more, I thought, Nice facility for a city of 28,000. Later, seeing the Paducah Medical Center and nearby Western Baptist Hospital I thought in terms of overkill.

In the downtown area I paused to take a picture of the weary old Irvin S. Cobb Hotel, named after the city's well known humorist and writer who died in 1944. He's the guy who said, "I'd rather be born in Paducah than be natural twins in any other city in the world." I took the picture as a souvenir for my son, Mark, who has read some of Cobb's books and enjoyed his humor.

Paducah, which calls itself the Gateway to Kentucky's Western Waterland, boasts of its recreation facilities, its festival events, performing arts, museums and other tourist attractions. And deservedly so for a city of 28,000.

On the negative side, the downtown area appeared to be in dire need of revitalization. I smiled when thinking, if I looked as tired as downtown Paducah, I'd be immobilized.

Seeing some of the manufacturing centers in the Paducah area, I was reminded of a conversation last night with the manager of the RV park. I had said something about horses and whiskey being important to the state's economy and he had replied, "Oh, they're big contributors all right – and they get the most notice. But the fact is manufacturing and agriculture are more the base of the economy. Just as one example, the area you're in, western Kentucky, produces two-thirds of the country's burley tobacco."

"Well, that's state number 29," Elaine commented when photographing me on the bank of the Ohio River. "But like Robert Frost said, 'Miles to go before we sleep'."

"You know," I said, "I've been thinking. I've been here three days in the state that is the world's biggest producer of bourbon and famous for its Kentucky fried chicken, and I haven't tasted either. I must be a spoil sport or party pooper, or whatever."

"So what's new," she replied. Again no respect.

All told, as I thought back on it, Kentucky was easy pickins'. I escaped both Highway 45 and Mayfield without any encounters. Running conditions on Highways 97 and 121 were above average, and excellent on Highway 45.

All body components functioned smoothly. The only problem was one stormy day, thunder and lightning in the background, which I survived with nothing more than a drenching. Yep, easy pickins'.

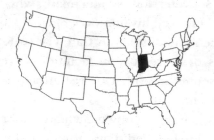

Chapter 3

Indiana

Cutting a Corner and Regretting It

Dates: *May 4th and 5th, 1997*
Miles: *27.5*
Route: *Start on bank of Ohio River, Illinois-Kentucky border, in Evansville near Angel Mound State Historical site. North in city to Highway 62, then follow 62 west to Wabash River and Wabash Memorial Bridge, Indiana/Illinois border.*

DAY ONE. "The adventure of running across states has to be fun, but the writing you do about it sounds like a lot of work. Are you sure it's worth all the work?"

These words, recently spoken by a running friend, came to mind as once again I set about to write about a state, groping for a way to begin and then laboring through the chapter. From time to time I do have to remind myself that it is worth all the effort, the time, the frustration.

Not that I am producing anything of literary merit, for I am at best a pedestrian writer. Rather, the merit of my story is the positive influence it has on some people.

I've had younger people say, "Seeing what you have done has influenced me to keep exercising." Some older folks have said, "After reading about your running, I decided to increase my walking program and I've been surprised at what I've been able to do."

But the most encouraging words I've ever had from readers have come from two blind people who had listened to the Library of Congress recording of *Ten Million Steps*.

Ruth Finis, a lady from Grapevine, Texas, phoned to say, "I just had to call and let you know how much I enjoyed your book. I can't tell you how much it has done for me." Ruth, a former teacher, now in her 70s, has been blind since age 52.

Rod Lawson, of Bellaire, Texas, wrote, "I'm one of your blind readers, and I can't tell you how much I enjoyed your book about your run across America."

The highest form of flattery I've ever had came form Bernie FitzGerald, of Hamilton, New Zealand, who told me he'd read *Ten Million Steps* a half-dozen times. Bernie, in his mid-60s, had to abandon running a couple of years ago when a knee gave out on him.

In early 1997 Elaine and I made the 135-mile drive from our home to San Francisco to meet Bernie and his wife, Jackie, who were visiting there. Meeting and visiting with them made the trip well worthwhile.

Another friendship formed after his reading of *TMS* was with John Cates, then Executive Director of the (California) Governor's Council on Physical Fitness and Sports, chaired by Arnold Schwarzenegger. In promoting physical fitness, John gives generously of his time and talents.

He was kind enough to nominate me as a consultant to the Council, and Arnold and Governor Pete Wilson approved the nomination. Attending the Council meetings has been an education for me.

The point of all this digression is that I don't have to flog myself to write as long as I remember the pleasant fallouts that ensue.

And so onward with Indiana. My original plan for running across the state called for running west to east across the southern part of the state, about 120 miles. That plan got torpedoed when the Indiana Department of Transportation (INDOT) sent me a list of roads on which pedestrians are prohibited, and my route was one of them.

At the same time I was told, "INDOT can only recommend a route that is best for your needs and purposes, and not grant approval for use of any particular roadway." The route that INDOT recommended was 280 miles, a bit over ambitious for what I had in mind.

INDOT stressed, "Any road travel will be at your own risk." And to make sure I knew the rules, INDOT sent me 12 pages of applicable statutes.

Well, at least, I had to give the bureaucrats credit for replying to my query about running across Indiana. That's more than some states did.

This reply left me searching anew for a route across the state. I had two choices: a route (north-south) of 200-plus miles or a route of less than 30 miles from the southern boundary (Kentucky) to the western boundary (Illinois).

While I would have preferred an east-west or north-south crossing, I elected this south-west one. One reason for doing so was that I was shaky about being able to complete 19 more states, so I took the easy way out.

If I had known how well I would hold up – by way of body and time frame – I would have chosen the longer route. The only consolation was that I did go across the state from the border of one adjacent state, Kentucky, to the border of another adjacent state, Illinois.

The route I hit upon started on the bank of the Ohio River in Evansville, the Indiana/Kentucky border, at Evansville, and followed Highway 62 west to the Wabash River , the Indiana/Illinois border. The distance turned out to be a mere 27.5 miles. We split these miles into two days, 19.2 miles the first day, and a shorter day of 8.3 that would give us an early start on our drive to Vermont.

The first day, a Sunday, took us from the Evansville environs to the eastern outskirts of Verona. The scenic highlight of the day was the passage through the waterfront area.

Evansville has one of the most beautiful landscaped riverfronts I've seen in any state. Much of it is bricked. It is a serene and immaculately kept companion to the adjacent Ohio River.

On the eastern end of this stretch of a half-mile or more are a number of mansions, all stately and of venerable vintage, overlooking the river. Sitting somewhat solitary in the middle of this parkway is the modern Azar Hotel and in the river across from it the City of Evansville riverboat, Indiana's first riverboat casino that offers the ultimate casino experience on the Ohio River.

The boat is a three-decker with Las Vegas-style entertainment and seven cruises every day. In other words, citizens, prepare to shed your shekels!

I talked with only one person all day, and this was early in the morning as I was easing out of Evansville. Cutting through a parking lot, I went past a guy standing beside his pickup which was towing a boat.

"Nice looking boat," I said by way of greeting.

"It gets me there," he replied. "Or it will if my friend ever shows up." I guessed him to be in his mid-50s. He was wearing sneakers, denim trousers and a T-shirt with a wolf and the words "I'm ready to howl" on the front of it.

Commenting on nobody else being around, I said, "Looks like we're the only ones out and about this Sunday morning. Everybody else must be in church."

I was hardly prepared for the barrage that followed: "I've got no use for organized religion. Most of it is built around fund raising and making money.

"Well, in fact, it goes way beyond that – I don't believe in religion or after-life. I believe you're put here but once. This is the only show in town, and when it's over, that's it for you. When the lights go out, you go out."

I said, "I'm sure there are a lot of people that feel that way, that there's no life after death. What I don't understand, for one thing, is if they think there is no accountability after death, why are they still such law-abiding citizens?"

"You mean," he replied, "if you believed there was no reward or punishment after you died that you'd not be a law-abiding citizen?"

"Well, for sure," I told him. "I'd be tempted to cut a lot of corners. I really don't know how far I'd go."

"I can say it's not morality that keeps me on the straight and narrow," he answered. "I'm not sure what does. Might even be a fear of getting caught and imprisoned.

"Might be the thought that there'd be anarchy if we didn't have respect for the law. Be a damn jungle out there. Might even just be that I like people."

I asked, "Do you feel that believing it's all over when you die makes life easier or harder for you?"

"Oh, a lot easier," he said. "I don't have a mess of religious hang-ups, and I don't have to fret and stew about what's going to happen to me after I die. Sure, I'd like to envision going on to some eternal paradise, but that's fairy-tale stuff."

"You seem pretty firm in your beliefs," I told him. "Think there's a chance that you might ever change your mind?"

"Well, I haven't in the past 30 years," he replied. "And it doesn't seem likely now. Ain't trying to convert me, are you?"

"No way," I said. "That would be the blind leading the blind. I'm still trying to sort it all out myself. One thing for sure, though, I certainly do believe in God, and to me it follows that if He exists so does some sort of life after death."

"Well, one thing for sure," he concluded, "this is one thing each one of us has to handle for ourselves."

Departing, I left him with these words, "I'll buy that. Take care now."

As I moved on, I thought it a mite ironic that, though we were not in church today, we were probably thinking more about religion than many people in church parroting hymns.

The only unusual incident of the day happened when, roadside, I found a Visa card, a phone card, and Blockbuster card – all evidently jettisoned from a stolen wallet. All were valid cards with an expiration date of 1998. After consulting a couple of phone books at one pit stop, Elaine and I found a way to mail them back to the owner.

Elaine reported that nothing unusual happened to her and the dogs today, although while she was walking them in one area a lady did remark, "They certainly seem to be well fed!"

Running on Highway 62 with its four divided lanes today was safe but also, like 45 in Kentucky, somewhat sterile. Once out of the Evansville area, I had no people or places contacts. I did have bad luck with the wind since it was a headwind all day.

Forestation lined both sides of the road. Beyond the forests the crops in this delta area were soy beans, wheat and corn.

This was another one of those days when, after finishing, we had to drive 30 miles to the nearest RV park.

DAY TWO. The temperature, in the low 40s, as we started our second day was a facsimile of our first day. Starting, I was not too sure of how I'd fare this day because at four A.M. I'd experienced another asthma episode, one that lasted 40 minutes and during 10 of which I was concerned about surviving.

We started on Highway 62 on the eastern edge of Verona and finished at the Wabash River, 8.3 miles west. Except for the passage through Verona, Highway 62 today was only two lanes. My running space consisted of two feet of pavement outside the fog line and two feet of gravel beyond this two-foot bike lane.

The last four miles or so were on a levee road, guard rails on both sides, extending through a delta area, much of it flooded. The trees protruding from the water reminded me of a Louisiana bayou.

Started on a couple of negative notes this second day in Indiana. After the early morning asthma episode, I was still struggling to get restored to normal breathing and I had the dry heaves.

The second negative was discovering that somewhere along the way our TV antenna was damaged by hitting a tree. Every bit as important as the money consideration would be the time and effort spent locating a place to get it repaired.

Almost immediately after starting I was into Verona, a city of 7217, which from what I saw did not appear that big. I had to detour from Highway 62 in order to get a look at downtown Verona that sits perpendicular to the highway.

The centerpiece was the town square with the county courthouse smack in the middle of it. A marble plaque on the yard there caught my eye and, reading it, I saw it was a list of the Ten Commandments. I found myself thinking, whatever happened to the separation of state and church?

My other reactions while passing through Verona were these:

- Another one of those cities in which, zoning absent, residences and businesses are interspersed.
- What economy supports the beautiful homes on the western edge of the city, homes that in California would sell for half a million dollars?
- Seeing a Subway franchise, I got the impression that we've not gone through a town, regardless of how small, that does not have a Subway franchise.

Leaving Verona, I found the two-lane road a big comedown from the comfort and safety of yesterday's breakdown lane. The light traffic, as well as knowing that I had only 8.3 miles to go, made conditions tolerable.

Other than for the annoyance of the asthma, I had no problems. At times I found myself wishing I had selected a longer route across Indiana, especially one that would have afforded opportunities to meet people.

Francis Bacon once said (and I know this from having to read his essays as part of a college course!), "Some books are to be tasted, others to be swallowed, and some few to be chewed and digested." I felt that at best I was only tasting Indiana; I would have preferred some swallowing.

Couldn't help thinking this morning of the conversation yesterday with the guy who said he had no use for organized religion. Interesting, as I've found out on more than one occasion, how a person will suddenly and impulsively unload details of his personal life to a stranger. I'd bet that many of the guy's friends don't know how he feels about religion.

From what I was seeing – agriculture and little else – the folksy, homespun Hoosier image seemed quite appropriate. But I realized this was not the full measure of the state which has areas saturated with automotive plants and steel manufacturing to such a degree that agriculture, big as it is, is only the state's second-largest contributor to the economy.

Just as the economy contrasts (agriculture and manufacturing), so does the folksy Hoosier image with the achievements of some native sons. As but one example, the sophisticated lyrics of Cole Porter and Hoagy Carmichael, both native sons, are hardly homespun stuff.

Once I left Verona and all the way to the finish at the Wabash River, the only distraction along the road was the Weilbreen ostrich farm, three miles west of Verona. Whenever I see these birds, I recall what a tour guide told me in South Africa: They're not very smart, with brains only the size of a walnut, and they mate for life. These, like others I've observed, were fleet of foot.

A couple of times on the CB radio today Elaine heard truckers say, "That old man on the road looks like he lost something."

Wrong, fellows. The reason the old man had his back turned to you was to prevent the dust and rocks you stir up from hitting him in the face and eyes. You guys have no idea of what stuff flies out from your truck's wheels and load. I was banged a few times before I learned to turn my back.

Coming to the finish at the Wabash River, I saw that the Memorial Bridge there was no youngster, dating back to 1955. The toll fees were reasonable enough, too, to date back a few years: 50 cents for cars, 75 cents for dual tires and 25 cents for each extra axle.

The toll keeper was not too enthusiastic about giving me permission to jog out to the middle of the bridge that marked the boundary between Indiana and Illinois. Elaine, who was parked in the toll lot, snapped a picture of me on the bridge and that was the full extent of our celebration over finishing Indiana.

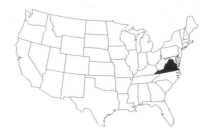

Chapter 4

Virginia

Following the Trail of the Lonesome Pine,
or Where I Was Baptized into the
U.S. Marine Corps

Dates: *May 7th and 8th, 1997*
Miles: *28.9*
Route: *Start in Kentucky on Highway 421, and follow it southeast to Virginia and Highway 352. When 352 intersects with Highway 70, follow 70 south to Tennessee border.*

DAY ONE. "Get your hands out of your pockets, you damn civilians!" That was my introduction and welcome to Virginia back in 1941 (good Lord, has it really been 56 years ago!) when, with a trainload of other officer candidates, I debarked from a train at Quantico to begin Marine Corps officer training.

Looking around, I saw that the order was barked by a sergeant wearing a name tag that read "Catalano." As I was thinking, This guy reflected a Marine Corps recruiting poster, he yelled another order, "Fall in!" The command was foreign to me and I wondered, What the hell do I do now?

And so began a three-month struggle to survive officer training. Little did I realize at that moment how much I would come to admire that same Catalano who labored so valiantly to mold me into a Marine.

Today I had considerably more confidence, despite my venerable vintage of 80, in surviving the run across Virginia than I did in 1941 of surviving officer training. And today as I started the run, the greeting, as contrasted with 1941, was somewhat warmer - a sign reading "Welcome to Virginia" and near it a plaque honoring Daniel Boone. Otherwise the starting scene on Highway 421 at the Virginia/Kentucky border was rather nondescript.

One reason that I exuded confidence today was that our route across the state was just an over-grown marathon, rounding out around 29 miles, which I decided to split into two days of running - the first, 14.5 miles, and the second, 14.4 miles.

It didn't require a lot of map study to see that the shortest route across the state was a north-south in the narrow southwest corner of the state. This route would begin on Highway 421 at the Virginia/Kentucky border, go southeast to catch Highway 58, and then connect with Highway 70, following it to the Tennessee border.

While Virginia travel books and tourist brochures speak glowingly of the state's attractions - Chesapeake Bay, sandy beaches, James River plantations, Shenandoah Valley, Blue Ridge and Allegheny Mountains, and many historic sties - not a word do they mention about the area we chose for our adventure. We were off the beaten path in Virginia.

Before starting, I knew - on the negative side - that the price I would pay for this short route was the risks of running a narrow, mountain road with blind curves and - on the positive side - there would be the variety of small towns, rural roads, fast-flowing streams and beautiful mountain scenery. Besides I was treading on history because Confederate and Union soldiers had used this route during the Civil War, so a series of historical markers told me.

Most of the road was through a gap in the mountains, covered with heavy tree growth that often extended to the very edge of the road. By my estimate none of the mountains was higher than 2500 feet. The few flat spots that did exist in the gap were occupied with homes, most of them substandard housing.

Because the road had no bike lane, I spent considerable effort and energy today when jumping from the road onto the grass whenever oncoming cars approached me. On some occasions when the other road lane was barren of vehicles, I could move to that side to avoid oncoming cars. I was able to do this most of the time when the coal-bearing trucks of the Gemstone Mine approached me, mainly because I had lead time since I could hear the grinding of their engines as they roared uphill.

What I remembered most about going through the two small towns – Stone Creek and Pennington Gap – was the heavy police presence in the form of sheriff and Highway Patrol cars. This, associated with the "no trespassing" signs on many homes, led me to believe this was a high crime area.

Remarkable, I thought as I passed a high school on the southern edge of Pennington Gap and saw it had an all-weather track. I wondered, How can the locals afford this facility? I took a 10-minute time-out to watch a track meet in progress.

The strongest impression of the day was seeing a hound dog fenced in a back yard. His area was built in a damp, muddy piece of ground.

To keep him out of the water and mud, the owner had built him a platform, about six by six feet, five feet off the ground. A dog house and water bucket sat on the platform, one-third of which was covered with his droppings.

Not much of a life spending countless hours on that platform, I thought as I saw the dog sitting forlornly there. Somebody once said something to the effect that to every dog his master is Napoleon. I doubted if this pooch felt that way.

Sort of found myself thinking, Wish I could bring Brudder and Rebel to this scene and say, "See, you guys, what an easy life you have!"

Only person I talked with today was a supervisor with a highway department team that was stopping trucks for a brake inspection. "What does vascar mean?" I asked him since I was curious after seeing a sign, "Speed checked by vascar".

"That's where they check you from point A to Point B," he told me. "That's all it stands for." Curiosity satisfied.

When I stopped to take a picture (damn Ansel Adams on the loose!) of a swinging bridge, the bridge revived memories of when I was in the first grade and had to cross one like it on my way to school. Living with my aunt and uncle at the time, I walked about four miles through the woods, then crossed the Russian River on a swinging bridge to get to school.

There were stories told in those days about a wild man who inhabited the area, and walking to school in the morning I was petrified with fear. For some reason I was not scared when I returned home in the afternoons.

The stories proved true because years later the man was captured and taken to University of California, Berkeley, for study. If I recall correctly (hey, don't bet on it these days!), a book was written about him.

The most exciting moment of the day happened when I stopped to adjust the belt of my fanny pack and, zowie, I became a high jumper when I saw a snake wiggling along between my feet. All I noticed as I reached for the stars was a fast-moving snake with a tan stripe down its backside.

This is, indeed, the South, I told myself when at one turnout I saw 15 dumpsters. In all the southern states I've run, dumpsters have been located at road junctions and turnouts.

This system of garbage disposal, like so many other systems, would be efficient and economical if people used it properly. But many don't because they fail to deposit all their garbage in the dumpster, and instead just toss it in the general direction of the dumpster. As a result the site becomes strewn with garbage.

Damn Navy captain, I muttered, almost as a conditioned reflex, when a pickup hauling a rattan couch and chair passed me. The rattan unleashed memories of a Navy captain who, returning from the Philippines, had completely filled the troop commander's quarters with rattan furniture he had purchased.

As the troop commander of a 1600-man Marine Corps task force returning to Oahu from a maneuver in the Philippines I had looked forward to the first time experience of occupying the spacious troop commander's quarters on a Navy transport. Upon reporting aboard, I was disappointed to be assigned to a cubbyhole stateroom and later ticked off when I learned the reason that I was not assigned to the troop commander's quarters.

The second day on board I got a small measure of retaliation when the captain asked if I would assign some men to do some chipping and painting on the ship.

"Ordinarily, Captain, I'd like to help out," I answered, "but these men are exhausted from being in the jungle for 45 days and nights. They need R & R." Saying no to a Navy captain on his kingdom afloat was very satisfying.

On both Highways 421 and 58 I had some roadside "mall" shopping at six different turnouts. Some locals had set up flea markets in the small, flat areas.

Our day ended on the familiar note of having a long drive, 28 miles in this case, to the nearest RV facility. It happened to be Stone Gap State Park, a pleasant introduction to the Virginia state park system.

DAY TWO. We started on Highway 58 in front of the Hillcrest Bowling Lanes, two miles north of Jonesville where we would connect with Highway 70 south. Jonesville prides itself on being chartered in 1794, and entering town I did, verily so, genuflect out of respect for such vintage, a good deal of which was reflected in the town's many old buildings. I also saw a number of empty store fronts leading me to ponder, Could there be a new Wal Mart nearby?

Seemed strange that a hamlet like Jonesville would have parking meters, but there they were. Here, as in Pennington Gap, I was surprised to see so many attorney offices.

Sort of a far cry from a Virginia law of 1658 that "expelled all attorneys from the colony." Speaking of attorneys, the county court-house in Jonesville suffered in comparison with most other county courthouses which are the centerpiece of the town.

Once out of Jonesville and onto Highway 70 – another of those roads with no bike lane and the fog line bordering on the grass shoulder – I played hopscotch much of the way when jumping from the road to the grass to avoid oncoming cars. Besides being curvy, 70 had some hills of a mile or longer with seven – and eight-percent gradients. The going was tough; the mountain setting, beautiful.

The most unexpected sight of the day happened early morning when I saw 20 or more buffalo grazing on a hillside. So unexpected were they that I had to look twice to make sure I was seeing buffalo.

They resurrected memory of an historical marker I once read. Rarely have I read anything that told as much as this marker of what the buffalo meant to the Plains Indians. It read like this:

"The buffalo was the department store of the Plains Indians. The flesh was food, the blood was drink, skins furnished wigwams, robes, blankets and beds, dressed hides supplied clothing and moccasins, hair was twisted into rope, rawhide bound tools to handles, green hide made pots for cooking over buffalo chip fires, hides from bulls' necks made shields that would turn arrows, ribs were runners for dog-drawn sleds, small bones were awls and needles, from hooves came glue for feathering arrows, from sinews came thread and bow strings, from horns came bows, cups and spoons, and even from gall stones a 'medicine' paint was made. When the millions of buffalo that roamed the prairies were exterminated, the Plains tribes were starved into submission."

On top of one ridge line today I stopped to talk with a truck driver who was parked there. "What kind of wildlife is there in this area?" I asked.

"Just about everything," he said.

"You mean bears?"

"Oh yeah, and some coyotes. Once in a while a mountain lion."

In my book, mountain lions are like the lotto. Only takes one to do the trick. The guy made me glad I was seeing no wildlife.

Today, as yesterday, at intervals I saw plaques reading "Trail of the Lonesome Pine." I assumed they had to do with the enormously popular book of that title published in the early 1900s. Though I had read the book in my youth, I could make no association with plot, setting or characters.

The day not being unusually warm, I was tempted not in the least to pause for a swim in the Powell River when I crossed over it. As I looked northward from the bridge, the river with trees to both edges looked like a postcard scene.

A shaky reaction when five dogs suddenly appeared on the road 50 yards ahead of me, but it lasted only momentarily because they exuded friendliness.

It's said that a dog laughs with his tail. That so, these guys were practically in hysterics. I regretted not having a handout for them because they all appeared to be in need of a hearty meal.

The two most interesting structures today were one that reflected opulence and the other, decadence. The opulent one was a mansion of the Civil War type so often depicted in Hollywood movies: two stories, columns and veranda in front, and three chimneys on the roof. It seemed out of place in this rural setting, yet it has been a landmark along this road a century or more.

The decadent one was a decaying cabin, along with a barn and out-house, located in a gully. I was hard put to understand why they were located there with drainage from three hillsides flowing toward them.

Going along, I noticed that the homes and yards on Highway 70 were much better maintained than those on 142 and 58. Why, I did not know.

I also noticed that not one of the more than a half-dozen farmers, guys in their 50s and 60s, driving pickups returned my friendly wave – whereas all the women did. Why, in this case, I did know, but being the modest type, I will let the reason go unspoken!

Around the end of this day I found my legs were lobbying for a rest. I suspected that the tiredness was not so much from running but from all the effort exerted jumping from the road onto the grass to avoid oncoming cars. The stop-go action was tiring physically and agitating emotionally since the energy expended does not move me forward.

But I have come to recognize that with recent states I have mellowed considerably in dealing with oncoming traffic. Nowadays when a vehicle approaches, I maneuver to get out of its way, whereas in my early days of state running, I'd challenge the driver, hold to the road to the last minute trying to induce him to move over. And if he didn't move over, I usually fired some naughty language in his direction. These days I have ceased and desisted such action because I consider it a waste of energy and I need all the energy I can muster.

I was not sure which was the more unexpected along Highway 70, seeing so many homes, one about every quarter-mile, or seeing no wildlife in this mountain setting. Highway 70 was different from 421 and 58 in that I saw no agriculture along it until the last three miles or so when the gap widened to a small valley. My general impression of 70 was that I was either going up or going down.

When, around 11.5 miles, I came into a small valley, about a half-mile long and 600 yards wide, I sensed that I was approaching Blackwater though no signs were about. This was confirmed when I came to the junction of Highways 70 and 604 and saw a store which served as the local post office, gas station and grocery. The valley, with 10 homes scattered about it and a stream flowing through it, was bracketed on all sides by mountains.

Shortly out of Blackwater I came across two Bell Atlantic employees, Ronald McFarland and Bill Myers. "What'cha doing out here?" Ron asked me.

"Well, at this point, I'm close to finishing a short run across your state," I said.

"Where'd you start?" Bill asked.

"On Highway 421 at the Kentucky border."

"That's a pretty good distance," Bill answered.

"Speaking of distance," I said, "how far is it to the Tennessee border?"

"Somewhere between two-and-half and three miles," Ron told me.

In those remaining miles, as the valley channeled toward the Tennessee border, I saw the only agriculture that appeared along Highway 70. I also went past the most modern structure seen since I started Virginia, this being the Sarepta Baptist Church, a new brick building at the junction of Highway 610.

I was momentarily puzzled when I saw 30 or so cars parked bumper to bumper. The situation became clear when I saw a hearse parked in front of a home.

Vividly into my mind flashed memories of a collateral duty I had when I was executive officer of the Navy ROTC unit at the University of Missouri in Columbia. Whenever Navy or Marine Corps personnel were killed in our area, I had to make a condolence call to the family and make sure they were receiving all the benefits and services to which they were entitled.

My first such call was a shocker because, entering the home, I learned that the custom was to have the casket and body in the living room for relatives and friends to view. The body, the crying, the sobbing did not make for a pleasant experience.

There was nothing distinctive about the Tennessee border except for the sign that told us we had arrived there. We could not celebrate our Virginia finish with a treat of some sort because we finished in the hinterlands with creature comforts far removed.

Virginia now history, we drove to Kingsport, Tennessee, and positioned ourselves to run that state. Overnighting at a KOA off I-81 in Kingsport, we studied three possible routes across Tennessee.

We went to bed undecided about whether or not to scout each one of them or to simply take off on one of them tomorrow. Who knows, we might even be following in the footsteps of Davy Crockett, or have I got that right? He was from Tennessee, wasn't he?

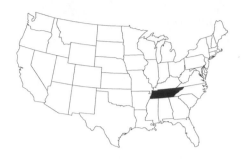

Chapter 5

Tennessee

In the Footsteps of Daniel Boone

Dates: *May 9th and 10th, 1997*
Miles: *22.8*
Route: *Start in Virginia on Highway 91 a quarter-mile north of Virginia-Tennessee border. Follow 91 south to 421, then take 421 south to North Carolina border.*

DAY ONE. As I was finishing Kentucky and contemplating Tennessee, up by association popped Davy Crockett's name – and then almost immediately I was questioning my sometimes fuzzy memory asking, Was Davy Crockett actually from Tennessee? Yes, he was, I confirmed as I dipped into Tennessee lore before starting across the state.

But that business, as popularized in song, about his being "born on a mountain top in Tennessee" was pure bushwa. More factually he was born on the banks of Limestone Creek near Greenville.

Later, as I progressed across the state I learned that my Tennessee associations should have gone to Daniel Boone rather than to Davy because it evolved that our route would follow the Daniel Boone Heritage Trail across the state (albeit that Boone, traveling from North Carolina to Kentucky as he went through Tennessee, was going south to north compared to our north-south routing). Nowhere along our route was there mention of Davy Crockett.

It had taken but a quick look at a map for us to recognize that the key to the shortest route across Tennessee lay in the narrow northeast corner of the state. The question was: Which of two routes, both north-south, to follow – Highway 421/34 from Bristol to Trade and the North Carolina border, or Highway 91 from Damascus to connect at Mountain with 421/34 south to Trade and the North Carolina border?

The only way to know which route was better was to reconnoiter them. We decided to scout the Bristol route first.

Doing so, we had to drive through Bristol – that's Bristol, Virginia, *and* Bristol, Tennessee, because State Street, the main drag and road leading to Highway 421, is bisected by the boundaries of the states. Each side has its own city and government services.

The entire complex, comprising both cities, is an important industrial center. A tourist could easily drive through the area – say, down the middle of State Street – and not realize he was straddling two states. Speaking of straddling states, it was news to me that Tennessee borders on eight other states (which ties it with Missouri as being the state with the most other state borders).

Catching Highway 421 out of Bristol, we were not on it very long until we realized that it was inhospitable to running and horrendously curvy and mountainous for the motorhome. When we came to the junction of 421 and 91, after approximately 35 miles of travel on 421, Elaine proclaimed, "I don't want to take the motorhome over that road again."

Her proclamation put us in the position of having to reconnoiter Highway 91 north to see if it offered a feasible route. Our scouting mission, which concluded at the town of Damascus, Virginia, unfolded a road that contrasted dramatically and favorably with the northern part of 421 that we had just driven. Highway 91, extending from Damascus on the north to Mountain City on the south, was a flat road through a canyon or gap area. Easy decision; our route would start at Damascus, follow 91 south to Mountain City, then take 34/421 to the North Carolina border.

Before starting, we toured Damascus (a name that, because I could not recall from whence it came, frustrated me to the point where I had to make inquiry to learn that its namesake was Damascus, Syria – believed to be the oldest city in the world). The town, with its many facilities, appeared bigger than its population of almost 1000 would indicate.

The town's distinction is that five important trails converge on it – the Appalachian Trail, the Virginia Creeper Trail, the Iron Mountain

Trail, the Transcontinental Bicycle Trail, and the Daniel Boone Heritage Trail. Which explained why we saw so many hikers about town.

As I edged out of town, south on Highway 421, signs told me I was on the Daniel Boone Heritage Trail. In a short distance I came to the Tennessee border and an historical marker telling that the state was first settled in 1769.

Highway 91 had its good points and bad. On the good side, a beautiful passage through forested mountains shouldering both sides of the road and the company of a fast-flowing creek, Laurel Creek by name, cascading over rocks. The usual reaction of people seeing this creek today is probably, great place to swim, great place to boat, great place to fish.

I mused, how many realize what a lifeline this water was for pioneers: water to drink, water for cooking, water for washing and bathing, water for irrigation. Pioneer homes were located near water for such reasons.

On the bad side, Highway 91 was a two-lane road with the fog line at the edge of the grass, no bike lane, considerable traffic, plus having blind curves. To handle a blind curve safely requires that I cross to the other side of the road whenever I approach such a curve.

For example, if I am facing traffic and come to a blind curve to the left, I cross to the right side so I can be seen by traffic. The problem here is that I am at the mercy of cars descending on me from the rear.

Despite its bad points, Highway 91 was manageable for me – in fact, much like many other roads I've run. Besides, the distance along it was only 15 miles or so.

Only a couple of tourist attractions appeared along the route today, both shortly after five miles. One was the Russell Stowe home and farm dating back to 1840. The well-preserved home probably endured for two reasons: loving, tender care and being well built.

The other attraction was Crowder's Classic Cars where I saw a Mark IV Lincoln Continental in mint condition and made a mental note to return here and buy it as soon as I won the lotto. Amazing how that lotto wish-list keeps getting longer all the time!

Soon after I started today, a light drizzle began to fall. It kept mounting and climaxed into heavy rain, thunder and lightning by the time I had covered seven miles. The weather such, we followed our inviolate rule of not running during thunder and lightning. Because our reconnoitering and touring of Bristol and Damascus had resulted in an afternoon start, it was already mid-afternoon and time to stop anyway.

The best happening of the day was the Johnson County Welcome Center, only eight miles from our finish, operated a comfortable RV facility. There our motorhome was parked six feet from the edge of a bluff, 100 yards down from which was a stream of clear, fast-flowing water. The trick now was to make sure the motorhome did not roll over the edge and that the dogs did not scamper down the bluff for a swim.

DAY TWO. Before getting into this second day in Tennessee, let me digress to running shoes, about which I am often asked. One of my goals while running across 23 states this year is to do all the running in lightweight shoes, what the trade calls "racing flats."

I have with me six pairs of the same brand, same model, a shoe weighing eight ounces each. Six pair because, seeking all the protection I can get while keeping the shoe lightweight, I intend to wear no pair for more than 250 miles, a conservatively safe distance to make sure that the shoe does not break down.

Why wear racing flats? Basically because they require less effort than heavier shoes.

Let's say I wore 11-ounce shoes instead of eight-ounce. That would mean that with each step I'd be lifting three ounces more. Multiply three ounces by the number of steps in each day's run and it's readily apparent that many extra pounds are being lifted with the heavier shoe.

Reason two: I find running much more enjoyable in racing flats than in heavier training shoes. That's why I've trained and raced in racing flats the past 25 years.

The great New Zealand marathoner Jack Foster advised runners, "Wear the lightest shoe you can get away with." That's reason three: at 145 pounds and a light hitter (i.e., I don't pound the pavement), I can get away with racing flats all the time.

The particular racing flats I am wearing on this safari are the most comfortable and protective I've ever worn. Since naming the brand and model would be tantamount to an endorsement, I'll not name either.

Speaking of endorsements, as part of the planning for our USA run I tried to get a shoe company to sponsor me by anteing up $5000 to cover expenses of the run. I contacted all the major shoe manufacturers, including the one that spends millions for endorsements from name athletes.

The answers from all manufacturers were uniform: "We have read your proposal and find it interesting, but we are not interested. Good luck with your run."

One of my joys after finishing the 3192-mile USA run was that I was beholden to no sponsor. If I would have had one, some people might be inclined to think that I did the run for the money. On reflection, it turned out for the best that we marched to the beat of our own drummer.

One last word about lightweight shoes/racing flats: In them I feel closer to being barefoot, closer to the earth, which in the main is why I also don't wear socks while running. But that's another story.

A couple of positive thoughts as I started this morning. Lucky for me that the grass on this road shoulder has been mowed, as this helps me to see what's there when I infiltrate it—which oncoming traffic has forced me to do 90 percent of the way on this road. Sort of uplifting, too, to see a scenic stream, much of it white water, alongside me.

Very relaxing to come into Mountain City and have a sidewalk to run on as opposed to having to step off the road almost continually to avoid cars. The northern approach to Mountain City was beyond expectations: upper middle-class homes lining Highway 91, no fast-food joints, no businesses tainted this residential district.

I stopped to take a picture of a two-story brick home with an historical plaque in front of it. I learned that the house was built by Roderick Random Butler, who came to this county at age 14 to be an apprentice tailor.

He went on to serve as a lieutenant colonel in the 13th Tennessee Calvary in the Civil War, then later served 24 years in the state legislature before being elected to Congress. He completed this home in 1870.

Born in 1827, he died in 1902, which means by my math that he lived in the house 32 years. Reading the plaque, I had two afterthoughts: If this guy managed his troops as well as he designed and built this home, he must have been Napoleonese. And if this apprentice tailor rose so high, what stars did a journeyman tailor reach for and grasp?

I saw the name "Hines" on a mailbox and smiled as I thought back on Jimmy Hines. He sat in the first row of one of my classes in my first year of teaching.

I was trying to inject some humor into the day's lesson, and the response seemed better than I had hoped for. The kids were laughing, sort of looking at each other, some half-laughs, some giggles.

Just about the time I thought I was a smash hit, I noticed Jimmy pointing to a note he'd written and turned upside down for me to read, "Your fly is open!" Red-faced I turned around, wrote on the blackboard with my right hand and hoisted my zipper with my left.

As I turned onto Highway 421 at its junction with 91, signs again reminded me I was on the Daniel Boone Heritage Trail. Seems there's no getting away from you, Daniel.

The southern end of Mountain City reflected what I had come to consider as the standard approach to a small American town: fast-food joints, gas stations, tire stores, garages, car dealerships and all such.

Here's a sampling of how life is on the road. I asked four people in Mountain City, "How far is it to the North Carolina border?"

In a positive tone the first one answered, "Fourteen miles."

A gas attendant said, "Ten miles."

The third: "Well, you're looking at Boone 35 miles away. So I guess it must be 20. I really don't know for sure, though."

The fourth: "I think it's about halfway between here and Boone, but I could be wrong."

All four of these people were locals, all living close to the state line, and all were wrong. When I scaled out the map last night, I judged the distance from Mountain City to the North Carolina border to be 12 miles.

Considerably more traffic than I had expected to find on departing Mountain City. All four lanes, two in each direction, were jammed with traffic.

At the junction of Highways 421 and 67, I read a sign proclaiming this was Shoun's Crossroads, established in 1792. Nothing here now but a gas station, a lumber supply and a real estate office. In colonial days the area was the scene of much trading.

Passing a senior rest home, I pitied the folks residing there. Six chairs were on the front porch, and the only view from there was the passing traffic. Sort of a bleak area, no yard, no access to a walking area for these folks.

A thought about how we age crossed my mind as I went past this rest home. This thought has fascinated me every since I read about it recently.

How we age is mostly a matter of how we live. "Only about 30 percent of the characteristics of agingis genetically based; the rest, 70 percent, is not," reported the MacArthur Foundation Consortium on Successful Aging.

Following up on that theory, out here on the road playing kid, I should be turning back the clock. Damn, come to think of it, much more of this and I might be romping around in diapers!

Almost did a Pavlov drool when, a short ways south of Mountain City, I saw a huge plant with the sign, Sarah Lee Home Products. Visions of Sarah Lee coffee cakes and cheese cake danced in my head. I was thinking of invading the plant to get a Sarah Lee fix, but my high went flat when I read the fine print on the sign: Sarah Lee Knitted Products.

Half a mile down the road when I came upon a golf course, I noticed only four players on it this windy, chilly day. As I took in the course and clubhouse, I thought, rather elaborate setup.

Then I saw the name: Roan Valley Estates. Whoa, that rings a bell!

Seems that Daniel Boone was on a trip here when his horse, Roan, became lame and Boone is said to have released him in a beautiful fertile valley. Thus the name Roan Valley. Like the man said, Daniel, there's no escaping you.

As I went along, I could not get over the dramatic contrast between Highway 421 from Bristol to Mountain City and Highway 421 south of Mountain City to the North Carolina border. The Bristol 421 was horrendously curvy and hilly, whereas the 421 south of Mountain City was almost flat, with a few hills of three-percent gradient.

When I was less than eight miles from the border, Elaine heard one trucker tell another on the CB, "An old guy on the road asked me how far it is to the North Carolina border. You think he can run that far?" Once again, Elaine's cue to come on stage and tell what Father was doing.

No unusual sights in the last few miles today. The hamlet of Midway didn't show much, just a building that was a combination convenience store, grocery store, gas station and bar–sort of a community hangout.

Was left to wonder why bird houses are so popular in these parts when I passed the third place I'd seen selling them. Must say the selection was imaginative: a southern mansion bird house, a conventional bird house, a log cabin bird house, a country store bird house, just to name a few.

Signs of the times or signs of values, I guess, that some of the small homes along the way had TV dishes that seemed to be worth more than the house itself.

Near the end of the run a sign alerted me that I was entering "historic Trade." Historic in that the site was used as a barter site by Indian traders before settlement.

Later Daniel Boone (yep, him again!), James Robertson and other pioneers used the Trade gap. The gap was an area of open land, about a quarter-mile by a half-mile, and is one of the oldest settlements in Tennessee.

What I saw there were about 20 homes, an antique store and a flea market. The old Trade days wagon road is well marked and preserved and nearby is a small park.

On a Tennessee map Trade appears to sit directly on the border. But don't believe it because I was a half-mile south of Trade still searching for the border.

Then I spotted Elaine parked 600 yards down the road. Bingo, the border!

And so, if I may paraphrase Lowell Thomas (which takes me back almost 50 years), we bid fond adieu to Tennessee. We now had North Carolina on our mind. Sorry about that, Daniel.

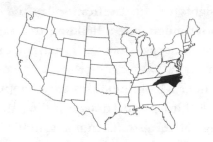

Chapter 6

North Carolina

DeSoto Beat Me Here

Date: *May 12th, 1997*
Miles: *20.4*
Route: *Start in Tennessee on Highway 68, which leads to Highway 294 in North Carolina. Follow 294 southeast to Highway 74. Take 74 north to 19/129 and follow 19/129 south to Georgia border.*

Easy was the decision about which of North Carolina's three major areas – mountain, heartland, coastal – to run across. The mountain area was the choice on several counts: its scenery, the attraction of the Blue Ridge and Great Smoky Mountains, and the short route across the western edge of the state.

The heartland area I rejected as being too long and the coastal area because it offered nothing new by way of sightseeing and because I had lived there for about two years on Marine Corps tours of duty. I do harbor a sentimental attachment to the coastal area inasmuch as my youngest daughter, Susan, was born there – at Marine Corps Air Station, Cherry Point.

Actually, as Elaine and I knew beforehand, the touristy attractions of the mountain area would come on the drive to and from our running route, and not so much on it. And so it was as, driving, we enjoyed the beauty of the Blue Ridge and Great Smoky Mountains, and saw such man-made attractions as the Biltmore Estate, Chimney Rock Park and the Grove Park Inn Resort.

Looking at the magnificent Biltmore Estate, a 250-room private residence, I thought, How in God's name can any person, no matter how rich, have the egoism and effrontery to build such a home? I thought of Chimney Rock as a reflection of American's focus on motorization – a great natural wonder where, for most visitors, the access is not by walking but by a 26-story elevator ride.

About the Grove Park Inn Resort, four years older than I, a huge complex built of native granite boulders and picturesquely nestled mountainside, I had but one thought: Elaine and I must return here sometime for a few vacation days and sojourn into neighboring Asheville, which we found to be every bit as attractive as advertised.

And so it was that we arrived at the Tennessee/North Carolina border on Highway 294 for our run across the state. Except for the border sign, the only distinctive feature about the spot was a farmer's barn that resided half in Tennessee and half in North Carolina.

The route we planned followed Highway 294 south to Highway 74, following it a short way east to connect with Highway 60 south. It didn't quite work out as such because Highway 60 was closed for construction, and in its place we had to follow Highway 19/129 to the Georgia border.

The whole jaunt, by our reckoning, was a mere 21 miles. It wasn't the pure north-south or east-west route we preferred, but it was across the state, so we settled for that.

Highway 294, a very narrow two-lane road with no shoulders, is such a backroad that it does not even appear on some maps. But the route has been around a long time because I had gone just a half-mile when an historical marker told me, "in 1540 an expedition of Spaniards led by DeSoto, the first Europeans to explore this area, marched out of North Carolina near here."

The question that crossed my mind: So marching, were these Spaniards wearing the body armor that all the history books show them wearing? If so, besides the weight, the armor should be a bit sticky and sweaty in the humid south. Might be useful, though, in fending off mosquitoes!

Elaine said, "No, mosquitoes are attracted to sweat." Score one for her!

The route was more hilly than mountainous, with very little cultivation but some cattle grazing in the open, grassy areas, of which there were few in this heavily forested area of mostly pine trees. Much of the way along Highway 294, I had the company of a fast-flowing creek of clear water. I was in a world far removed from urbanity.

Driving to the start, we had seen a number of loose dogs along the road, which made me a bit apprehensive. Getting underway, I saw a dog 100 yards in front of me, then he saw me and took off in the opposite direction at full speed. Relief!

At another point I was charging up a hill when I saw a German Shepherd and what I thought was a small dog coming toward me. Then, taking a second look, I said, "Hell, that's not a small dog, it's a goat."

Shepherds and Doberman always get my adrenaline pumping, but this guy heeded my, "Stay!" Which brings up the point that if I were limited to a vocabulary of one word, it would be "stay." It served me well today when dogs came out to the road to greet me or eat me.

The most exciting dog experience of the day was near a cabin where a guy had seven loose dogs. Two started toward me. I yelled "Stay!" but they were not heeding me.

About then from the cabin porch a guy, who looked to be in his early 50s and wore bibbed overalls and plaid shirt, roared a command to the dogs who ignored him. Whereupon, aiming in the general direction of the dogs, he fired a shot from the pistol he was holding. Instantly the dogs about-faced and raced frantically toward the back of the ramshackle cabin.

"That'll learn you to stay," he yelled. From his tone and the way the dogs reacted I got the impression he might have shot one on a prior occasion.

"Thanks," I said, "but they were probably wasting their time. I'm too gristly to be tasty."

"Oh, I don't know about that," he replied. "They like to chew on bones."

"In that case, I'm pretty ripe!" I said.

The cabin was one of the many residences, all spaced about a third of a mile apart, that lined Highway 294. Most of them were of modest means except for an array of luxurious homes about three miles from my start. I was at a loss to understand what these homes with all the creature comforts of urban sophistication were doing in this remote area.

I also couldn't understand why I saw no wildlife in this forested, hilly area. Home in our backyard in Auburn, California, Elaine and I see more wildlife than on this road. All day the only time I yelled "Wildlife!" was at 13 miles when a grasshopper jumped in front of me.

On a couple of counts I had difficulty adjusting to running today. The 250-mile drive yesterday did not help, nor did the fact that I was having breathing problems but fortunately no asthma attack.

There was a bit more traffic than I would have liked. I had to remind myself several times to be cautious because the natives drive with the fervor of a racing driver. It took me a while to adjust to all the passing pickups having their motors adjusted to be unduly noisy and roaring like a motorcycle.

It was amusing to see the bewilderment in the eyes of the natives as they passed me. Expressions saying, "What in hell is this?" Nice that they were friendly, most waving to me, even though they did not think of moving over to give me running room.

In addition to the company of the creek, I had the company of a heavy bird population, making their presence known by an almost continuous chirping. For all I know, they could have been warning each other: Watch out, the monster man is on the road.

The birds sort of reminded me of summer spent on my uncle's ranch in Depression times. I would be handed a .410 shotgun and 10 shells (a cost of five cents each), and told to come back with 10 birds so that my aunt could make a stew for dinner.

What kind of birds did not matter, but the number better be 10 or I would have some explaining to do. Kind of an interesting stew, by the way, with robins, blue jays, quail and unidentifieds.

My second conversation of the day was with Charles Holbrook. He had been sitting on his front porch watching the world go by when he saw me coming down the road and came out to talk with me.

His greeting sort of surprised me: "Well, you're a strange looking animal."

"I guess you don't see many ancient runners around here," I replied.

"You're a first," he answered. Hardly surprising, I thought, in Americana where a favorite retiree pastime, especially in the South, is occupying a rocking chair on a front porch.

Charlie went on to tell me that he has lived in this area since he was 10 years old, that he is now 67 (he looked a bit older, probably because he was toothless) and that he worked for the same factory in nearby Murphy for 35 years.

"I like this part of the country pretty good," he told me, "even though we get quite a bit of snow in the winter." As he spoke, I suspected he had not wandered very far outside of North Carolina.

I took leave of Charlie by telling him I had to hurry to Elaine, who gets worried if I am overtime. I needed an excuse to get away because Charlie who, for want of something else to do, was primed for an extended powwow.

Shortly after leaving him, going by a field I saw a calf so newly born that it could barely stand as it struggled to its mother for lunch. As it did, the mother looked at me, trying to read my intentions toward her child. I've had mothers do that before!

Couldn't help but think as I went along today how the runs this year, and I'm now into my sixth state, contrast sharply with previous state runs. Before, our runs were long with no days off.

This year we have a short run across a state, then get a day or two off driving to the next state. Now there's more of a vacation aspect.

The most memorable sight along Highway 294 was Fields of the Woods. Not knowing it existed, we were unprepared for it.

Elaine was parked in front of the huge cement archway with the inscription "Fields of the Woods." We could see a beautifully land-scaped driveway leading to the main facility.

I was thinking, What gives here? We took time out to investigate. After all, to quote my constant companion, "This is a vacation."

What we discovered was a 216-acre Bible park designed to memorialize the Church of God. It's an admission-free attraction filled with visitors during the tourist season. The only places to spend money are in the gift shop and restaurant.

As we drove into the park, the view was striking. On one grassy hillside, the Ten Commandants were spelled out in large white marble letters.

Atop another mountain was a 150-foot white cross. There was a replica of Golgotha and reportedly of the type tomb in which Christ was buried. Here, for some reason, it was called "Joseph's Tomb" on the driveway level, and on top of a telephone-sized metal tower with a cross in the form of a star, it was called the "Bethlehem Star."

The place – with its pavilion, gospel theater, picnic grounds, and nature trails–was intended for more extended visits than ours. For us, though, it was an interesting and informative diversion that added variety to our day.

About 13 miles into our day, and nearing the end of Highway 294, I came upon a white cross, beautifully decorated, and inscribed to the memory of Sarah Whitlock, age 15. One of so many white crosses I have seen marking highway fatalities.

How, on this clear, open road, did she die? Did she fall asleep? Did a careless driver come out from the side road and hit her? Did a drunk driver cause this?

When at 100 yards down the road I saw a young guy attending a brush fire, I wondered if I should ask him about Sarah. I was hesitant because maybe he was a relative and could be sensitive. I struck up a conversation with him and as a result learned a few things.

It turned out that he worked in the admissions office of Bennett College in Greensboro. Bennett, I learned, is a four-year college for black females.

It is one of two historic black female colleges in the USA. The other is Spellman in Atlanta.

Jene Keenum went on to tell me that Bennett's enrollment varies between 500 and 600 and that the prime majors there are pre-med, sociology, education and psychology. If I heard him right, it's a United Methodist college.

When I felt it safe to ask about Sarah, he told me hers was one of two fatal accidents in the area during the 94 years his great aunt has lived here. He said that Sarah came around the icy corner, her car slipped, then flipped, and the accident resulted in her death.

He told me that he was on a short vacation from his job and was visiting his parents, now retired, and helping to clean up around their place. He pointed to the house where he was born and said that, except for being away for schooling and now his job, he had lived here all his life.

"That's not very long, though," he said, "when compared to my 94-year-old great aunt who has lived here all her life."

He went on to explain that the family bought 140 acres here at a government auction after the government had taken the land from the Indians. Standing on the highway, I could look in a full circle and see most of this family acreage.

I suspected this land was part of the more than five million acres the Cherokee Indians lost through treaties with the U.S. government. Even though I'd read much American history, I'd never heard of the Cherokee plight and "Trail of Tears" until this summer when, on some highways, I saw plaques commemorating the infamous event.

Almost 14,000 Cherokee removed from their homes in Tennessee, Alabama, Georgia and North Carolina and forced to move, almost exclusively by foot, to arid Oklahoma. Along the way 4000 died of starvation, exposure and exhaustion.

A handful of Cherokee (a number estimated to be around 200) were able to hide out in North Carolina and avoid this Indian migration ordered by President Andrew Jackson, an Indian-hater. The town of Cherokee and the Cherokee Indian Reservation, both about 75 miles north of my running route, are a tribute to their survival. Their descendants reside on the reservation today.

Highway 74 was a pleasant interlude between 294 and 19/129 because it was a divided highway, two lanes each side and both with a bike lane. Unfortunately this pleasantry, the only relaxing running I had in North Carolina, lasted only two miles until I turned south on 19/129. As previously mentioned, I had intended to go south on Highway 60 to the Georgia border, but this road was closed for construction.

Highway 19/129 was nasty going from beginning to end. It was a narrow, curvy road–so much so that double yellow lines indicated no passing all the way. The fog line extended to the grass, and the shoulder grass was one foot high, so I never knew where I was stepping as I got off the road to avoid cars.

The traffic was practically bumper to bumper because the parallel road, Highway 60, was closed. I did not drink in the scenery or gawk around as much as I would have liked because I had to stay concentrated on approaching cars if I wanted to survive.

Actually there was nothing too distinctive to see during these last five miles or so. I do remember the road being dotted with flea markets and antique shops. Elaine and I both took note of the many wild red poppies alongside the road.

I vividly remember almost stepping on a snake, grayish-brown with orange horizontal stripes, and wondering, *what breed art thou?*

A highway department road sign was a first for me. It read, "Wipers on? Burn your lights."

As I did some day-dreaming in the last miles, my thoughts focused on some Marine Corps Commandants with whom I had crossed paths. Maybe this thinking was a fallout from having done two tours of duty, a brief one during World War II and a two-year stint in 1956-57, in North Carolina.

The first Commandant with whom I had a firsthand experience was Randolph Pate. He visited our unit in North Carolina, and our commanding general had ordered a briefing for him , saying, "And you damn well had better do a good job."

As a presenter I was a bit shaky about how I would come off. But it turned out I had naught to fear.

Pate nodded off during the briefing by the colonel before me. When he finished and the chief of staff nodded for me to commence, Pate was sound asleep and so he remained, much to my satisfaction, throughout my briefing.

The next Commandant I dealt with was David Shoup. Even before we met, there were things about him I did not understand:

- Why did he get a Medal of Honor at Tarawa? True, he planned the nuts and bolts of the tactical landing, but he performed no extraordinary heroic act. His life was no more in danger than the lives of many Marines around him.
- Why did he espouse physical fitness and weight control as a theme of his administration when he himself was 40 pounds or so overweight?
- Why, when he came to Japan to observe Marines there, did he bring his wife with him when by his very policy Marines ordered to Japan for 14 months were not allowed to bring wives or dependents, although the Army, Navy, Air Force personnel stationed there could and did?

My most severe criticism of General Shoup was reserved for his demeanor when he inspected a battalion I commanded in Hawaii. I introduced him to my sergeant major, Oscar Fargie, and said, "General, Sergeant Major Fargie was captured at Corregidor and spent the war in a Japanese prisoner of war camp."

Shoup's reaction was merely to brush the sergeant major off with a glance. I was pissed because in my book Fargie had suffered a lot more hell during his years as a prisoner than Shoup did during his few days on Tarawa.

In all fairness I could be misjudging General Shoup. After all, it's hard for me to understand a general who had a hobby of collecting tea cups.

When I attended Marine Corps Senior School (now known as the Marine Corps University), a future Commandant, Colonel Louis Wilson, sat directly in front of me. Wilson's major distinction was that he wore a Medal of Honor, one richly deserved for heroism in combat. I knew him only well enough to know that he was several cuts above both Pate and Shoup.

Near the end of my day, a first occurred when a gent with Georgia plates stopped to offer me a ride. I waved him on and, doing so, could not recall a prior offer of a ride in any other state so far this year.

The ending came suddenly today. Running down a hill, I saw Elaine parked by a sign with a historical marker, which I guessed to be the Georgia border. Nearby was a building with a lottery sign but nothing else distinctive – no river, no ridge line, no definite geographical feature.

The marker read, "The colony of Georgia was chartered in 1732, named for King George II of England, settled in 1733 and was one of the original 13 colonies."

If I remember American history correctly, most of the early settlers were convicts released on condition they migrate to America. No mention of that did I see.

Our short 20.4-mile crossing finished, we turned around and headed for West Virginia, which I estimated to be 450 miles away. As we started the drive, I asked Elaine, "Are you still having fun?"

"Very much so," she replied. "It would only be better if Randy Travis were sitting where you're sitting."

Damn, the lady calls it as it is!

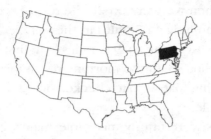

Chapter 7

Pennsylvania

The Lake Erie Connection

Dates: *May 16th to 18th, 1997*
Miles: *44.7*
Route: *Start on Highway 430, New York/Pennsylvania border, and follow 430 west to Highway 20, then take 20 west to Ohio border.*

DAY ONE. Some state runs – Montana, Oregon, Washington, Wyoming come quickly to mind – I remember fondly as labors of love. Others, because of some difficulty or deficiency, I remember mainly as devotions to the cause of running across all 50 states. My first two days in Pennsylvania fell into the latter category.

I blame myself more than Pennsylvania for this unhappy association. Had I listened to my friend David Prior, runner and attorney in Philadelphia, I might well recall Pennsylvania with fondness. David, hoping to ease my passage across the state, had recommended a route that was scenic, interesting and even shorter than the one I chose.

I didn't follow David's advice for a couple of reasons: First, his route brought us closer to metropolitan Philadelphia than we desired. Second, the route that we chose put us practically at the starting line of our next state (Ohio) to run, less than a five-mile drive.

Actually we even had to make a change in the route we had chosen to run, this being Highway 20 from the New York border west to the Ohio border. We were detoured from following the first dozen miles or so of Highway 20 because it was under construction.

Instead our route started on Highway 430 and followed it to its junction with 20, then we were on 20 the rest of the way across the state. All told, we ran only 44.7 miles in the state.

We were lucky to sneak in 9.6 miles our first day after a late afternoon start. We had spent the morning reconnoitering Highway 7 in Ohio, and following that we had checked out 20 in Pennsylvania to see if it was runnable.

These 9.6 miles were utterly miserable, mainly because the temperature was in the 30s and the wind was about 25 miles per hour. Weather forecasters rated the temperature as being in the 20s with the wind-chill factor. Kind of a dramatic adjustment for a fossil accustomed to running in temperatures ranging from the 80s to 90s.

Only a sign, no distinct landmarks, told me that I was at the New York/Pennsylvania border. The setting was agricultural, much cultivation, rolling hills.

Luckily the traffic was light on the two-lane paved road with a dirt shoulder. I had problems enough with the cutting wind; I ran hunkered and bundled.

Unlike me, Rebel and Brudder were having a great time experiencing gopher delight when Elaine walked them. It seemed that the dirt was soft, easy digging, the gophers were half-frozen, so the dogs were enjoying gopher hors d'oeuvres by the dozen.

The only laugh I had along the way was at the sense of humor of one farmer who had this sign on his front yard: "Snipe Farm. 10,003 caught last year. Hunting season now open for snipes."

This brought back memories of my high school days at a summer camp the Christian Brothers had on the Russian River near Guerneville, California. One of the favorite pastimes was to take the first-time campers snipe hunting and, by several types of trickery, to try to induce them to stay at this futile enterprise for hours.

DAY TWO. Pennsylvania produced the same unpleasant weather the second day as the first. On top of that I spent considerable effort dodging traffic.

The fact that my asthma was acting up did not help matters either. But I quit feeling sorry for myself when I passed a funeral home and saw people gathering for the procession. Once again I marveled at just being alive at 80.

There were a number of diversions along the way to help take my mind off running and, to some degree, the weather. The first was going past Penn State University, Erie, Behrend College. I saw a beautiful setting, green fields, buildings nestled against the forested mountains.

Penn State brought to mind legendary football coach Joe Paterno. I had but to close my eyes and could see him pacing the sidelines and exuding anxiety because his team was ahead by only 20 points.

I concluded that tax collector must be a good job in these parts because I saw political signs of five candidates running for just this one office.

Had to admire some kids from St. James High School who were having a car wash on this windy, cold morning. I also noted that St. James Catholic Church had six masses on Sundays and two on Saturdays, leading to the conclusion this area must be a Catholic stronghold.

Speaking of things churchly, a couple of unlikely neighbors: the Apostolic Church of Jesus Christ and the adjacent Steppin' Out Lounge.

Highway 20, going through Erie, reminded me of the Highway 80 we ran in Louisiana. Both were once main drags across the state until replaced by Interstates– in Pennsylvania, by I-90; in Louisiana, by I-20. On both routes, there were many reminders (motels, restaurants, etc.) of their having once been the main thoroughfare across the state.

The homes in east Erie were depressing. Maintenance and paint were foreign words.

The houses sat practically on the sidewalk. Where yard space existed, it was used for car parking. Porches and yards were strewn with litter.

Also depressing, for me at least, was to see the inordinate number of people smoking. I was definitely not going through one of the better areas of Erie.

Hands down, St. Vincent's Hospital was the most modern building I saw in Erie. Going past the Erie Veterans' Memorial Stadium, I peeked in and saw a bowl with an all-weather field and seating for about 20,000 spectators.

Evidence that high school football is big in the Keystone state. As I recall, Joe Montana, Terry Bradshaw and many other superstars had their origins in Pennsylvania.

All through the area, this still being east Erie, I saw a number of vacant store fronts. About a half-block of Highway 20 was a three-story plant, now out of business. A sign told me it had been a corset factory.

A major attraction for me was Bulakos, a candy store that has been in business for 92 years. I had no choice but to drop in and buy some chocolate fudge as a surprise for Elaine. Adherence to the maxim of Keep Thine Pit Crew Happy!

Couldn't understand why the vending machines were selling Coke and Pepsi for 35 cents, whereas the usual tariffs I've seen in other states vary from 50 to 60 cents.

Another thing I could not understand was why the Arthur Schultz Furniture Store, specializing in fine furniture and huge in size, extending one block, was located in a poor area of east Erie. Low overhead, Arthur?

The only extended conversation I had during my three days in the state happened in west Erie when I stopped by a store front to adjust my fanny pack. I was fiddling with the straps of the pack when I heard a guy saying, "I saw you coming down the sidewalk and I noticed your 'Running Across All 50 States' T-shirt."

Looking toward the source of the voice, I saw, standing in the entry to a jewelry store, a guy who reeked of prosperity. Expensive-looking clothes, tassel-adorned and highly polished loafers. He was smoking a cigar. I judged him to be in his mid-30s and in need of some exercise.

"Well," I replied, "you also probably noticed I wasn't moving very fast."

He said, "I was thinking if you're really running all the way across the state, you must have come from some place in the east near the Delaware River."

"Oh no, not quite," I told him. "I'm just running east to west from the Pennsylvania/New York border on Highway 430 to the Ohio border near Conneaut. Only about 45 miles and most of it on Highway 20."

To this he remarked, "I don't think I'd consider that across the state. It's only across a small part. 'Across' to me means the full length or width of the state. Do you shortcut all the states like this?"

"Not really," I said. "Until this year I was running the length or width of most of them. Like Kansas, which was 499 miles, or New

Mexico, 413 miles. But now I'm taking the shortest route across a state I can find."

"How come you're shortcutting them?" he persisted.

"Well, in a nutshell, I want to get across all 50 and I'm not so sure that I'll live long enough to be able to run the length or width of all those I have left to run."

Then he said, "I kind of noticed you are getting up in years. I'd guess you're almost 70. Right?"

"Pretty close," I replied. Why hurt his ego by telling him he was 10 years off. Besides, 70 rode smoother with my ego.

"Who's sponsoring you for this?" he asked.

"Nobody."

This surprised him. "You mean you're not getting any money? Nobody's giving you anything?"

"Not a penny."

"Then how come you're doing it?" he wanted to know. "What are you getting out of it?"

"By way of an answer, let me ask you, Do you play golf?"

"Yeah, some, but not very good," he said.

"Why do you play?"

"That's easy," he told me. "Because I have a good time. I enjoy it."

This was my cue to say, "And that's the same reason why I'm doing this."

"But wait a minute," he said, "it's not quite the same. Golf is play. What you're doing is a lot of work."

"Depends on how you look at it," I answered. "Kind of like sex. Some people consider that work. But most people do it because they enjoy it. And, by the way, these people aren't sponsored or paid."

That sex add-on just sort of blurted out, and I was surprised to hear myself saying it. Didn't hurt, though, because as he left to follow a customer into the store he was smiling.

Between talking with people and reading historical markers, I learned a bit about Erie. At the Eriez Campground last night, I learned that the Eriez were an Indian tribe wiped out by the Senecas and that Erie itself is named after the Eriez.

Historical markers told me that the city, laid out in 1795, is the only Great Lakes port in Pennsylvania and that the population is 108,718. It was news to me that Erie is the third-largest city in the state.

I had planned to do 19 miles my second day, but tired of the wind and cold and battling asthma I bugged out at 15.1 miles.

DAY THREE. The going was considerably easier today than the first two days. A nasty wind did persist, but the temperature rose to 70 degrees. The traffic was considerably heavier but tolerable because of a runnable shoulder.

The most distinctive sight of the day was St. Cyril Mehodius Catholic Church, one of the most eye-catching churches I've ever seen while running. It was an impressive stone building, about 400 yards off the road.

The first thing that caught my eye was a to-scale replica of Calvary. Next I saw a circular path with a number of stone pillars, each about six feet high. On second look I realized these were the stations of the cross around a grass field about the size of two football fields and divided by a road.

Later when I went past Holy Cross Church, doing a brisk business this Sunday morning, I realized I was seeing as many Catholic churches in these parts as I saw Baptist churches in the South. The churches and Sunday reminded me to follow my Sunday-on-the-road routine of dwelling a few moments on things religious.

One conclusion I have reached about religion at this stage in life is that there is no one true religion. They are all avenues, pathways to God.

If you believe in eternal life, religion is a crutch to keeping you moral. Religion is also a fortress in facing trials and tribulations of life. In World War II, a devout Catholic in those days, I was strengthened by religion as I faced the possibility of death.

The times, how they do change. In my youth, those early days in the Catholic Church and in a Catholic school, I savored the Latin liturgy of the church. I liked the tie-in with ancient times, with the advent of the church.

When in recent times the church went ecumenical, changing from Latin to English and introducing more singing and pomp, I was turned off by all the ceremonial jazz.

Other things, too, about the church have turned me off. An inspirational, interesting, relevant sermon from a Catholic priest is about as rare as IRS admitting it made a mistake.

And some teachings I cannot accept: that eating meat on Fridays or missing Mass on Sundays, both mortal sins, could get a person condemned to hell if he died unforgiven. I think it purely political that priests are not allowed to marry, arrogant that the church does not recognize valid grounds for divorce and intrusive that the church does not condone abortion in some cases. Enough, enough, I am bordering on excommunication!

Except for these reflections on religion, my mind today was pretty much focused on what I saw along the road. An array of sights and observations kept me occupied.

About the time I entered Fairview, a community of middle-class homes and some businesses, I unexpectedly came upon a big swampy area, almost a mile long, trees growing out of it, reminding me somewhat of a Louisiana bayou. Then, a bit down the road, another swampy area with a sign, "32 Acres for Sale." I didn't know what the buyer would use it for except to breed water moccasins!

Near the swampy area I saw a deer so big, almost the size of a colt, that at first I did not believe it was a deer. Seeing me, it said, "Good-bye, I'm outta here," and scooted away.

It's the political season, with all kinds of candidate posters about. Couldn't help but notice that at least 50 percent of the candidates have last names ending in "ski". Begorra, what chance does a poor Irishman have?

At the intersection of Highways 20 and 98 a donut shop carried a sign, "Closed on Sundays and Mondays." On *Mondays*? That's outrageous!

Both Elaine and I have noticed a change in driving habits here from the previous states run this year. These drivers are more aggressive, more stress-prone, less courteous.

Saw a couple of places called "Collision Centers" and stuttered over that awhile until I realized it was a euphemism for what out west, pardner, we call an auto body shop.

In sort of a reverie I went past a farm house and was rousted by the barking of a huge German Shepherd who seemed to be saying, "Hey, I haven't had lunch yet, old man. Wish I could break this damn rope and get at you."

In the center of the town of Girard I checked out a monument dedicated to Dan Rice, America's most famous clown of the 19th century who had winter quarters in Girard, 1823 to 1900. What mystified me was why would anybody in his right mind want to winter a circus in this frigid zone? Maybe if the old Girard Hotel in the middle of the six-block business district could talk, I'd get an answer.

Noticed that the residences in Girard, some big, most old, are very well maintained. Erie could take a lesson. Police are friendly, too; one gave me a wave and honk as he passed.

Scene on the road: from a farmhouse 100 yards off the road, a kid no older than five or six, drives a small battery-powered car up a dirt road toward the highway. There he turns around, returns to the house.

Some pluses and some minuses here. Plus: kid is happy doing something constructive, independent. Minus: a little danger of accident, more danger that the kid will grow up without exercise being a part of his life-style.

Another scene: A woman and her 16-year-old son cutting the grass of their yard, at least 150 by 150 feet. The son is riding a tractor mower, the mother is pushing a hand mower. Welcome to America, 1997.

Once again caught off-guard when I saw vineyards in this part of the country. Compared to the California vineyards, they all looked a bit puny.

Didn't feel very bright because of my confusion over boroughs, townships, towns, cities. Made a note to learn the distinguishing characteristics of each.

One way to describe my feelings today would be to say that I felt like a kid playing hooky from school. I was just out here, strolling along, taking in the sights, in a not-to-worry mood.

Pennsylvania was similar to some other states run recently: not a single offer of help or a ride and no police checking on us.

But there was one difference here: I found a dime, prosperity because it was more than the total money found in the six previous states.

This was not quite as good a deal as gotten by William Penn, who received the greatest land grant ever given an English subject. And what was Penn required to pay the king in return? Can you believe two beaver skins a year!

Reviewing Pennsylvania, I ranked the running as relatively easy and the weather as downright uncomfortable. In fact, I gained the impression that pleasant weather – the kind usually enjoyed in my area of California – is a rarity in the Lake Erie area.

While I was not nagged with any running injuries in the state, I did weather some asthma storms.

Pennsylvania finished, I took stock of where we were this year and found that we had completed seven states and had 16 yet to run. Let's see, that's just a whisker short of being one-third completed. Another refill, please, bartender, the party's just beginning!

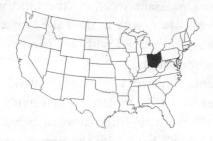

Chapter 8

Ohio

From the Shores of Lake Erie to the Shores of the Ohio River

Dates: *May 19th to 24th, 1997*
Miles: *102.6*
Route: *Start on shores of Lake Erie, near Harbour Marina, south on Park then Mill Street to connect with Highway 7 south. Follow 7 south to I-80 at Youngstown area, then take 616/630/170 south to 447. Follow 447 into East Liverpool and go through town to shores of Ohio River.*

DAY ONE. It was the Ohio River that caused us to switch running routes in Ohio. Originally we had planned to run across the state on Highway 20, but instead wound up running it on a different route. But I'm getting ahead of the story; back to the Ohio River.

The first time I saw the Ohio River – that being at Golconda the day I finished running across Illinois – I just stood and stared in silent awe. Never before had I realized that the Ohio was the source of so much power for industrialization. Seeing this magnificent marine super-highway, dividing line between North and South in the Civil War, made it easy for me to understand why this river played such an important role in western settlement and in 19th-century American commerce.

The second time Elaine and I crossed paths with the Ohio was in Indiana when I started my run across that state from Evansville on the river's bank. Once again I realized there had been a void in my geography lessons. I was never given to understand and appreciate this 981-mile river that flows northwest from Pittsburgh and then gradually southwest until it joins the Mississippi.

The Iroquois word for Ohio means "fine or good river." The Iroquois apart, I can't help but think of Japan every time I hear the word "Ohio" because a word pronounced as such (and spelled "ohayo") means "good morning."

When Elaine and I talked about our run across Ohio, we noticed that we would be able to see much of the Ohio River if we drove Highway 7 that paralleled the river from the southern tip of Ohio to East Liverpool, a distance of 185 miles or so. That would be a scenic drive of the river.

Then, studying the map, we realized that if we continued on Highway 7 all across the east edge of the state from East Liverpool to Lake Erie, we could scout this route and decide if it were feasible for a run across Ohio. What's more, if it were feasible, we could even tie this in with the run across Pennsylvania since a route there along Highway 20 from the New York border to the Ohio border would bring us very close to an Ohio starting point at Lake Erie.

Before the Ohio River got into the act, we were considering a route across Ohio suggested by Lou Abney, a Marine Corps classmate and attorney in Toldeo. Lou's suggested route, west to east mainly along Highway 20, was scenic with a number of attractions. Our only concern with it was that we would have to navigate through metropolitan Toledo, an adventure that thrilled neither Elaine in the motorhome nor me on foot.

The clincher in jettisoning Highway 20 and in favor of Highway 7 as our running route was our scouting mission as we drove Highway 7 from south to north. We liked the countrified setting, light to moderate traffic, sufficient camping and no metropolitan areas to negotiate.

The next step was to devise a battle plan. We estimated the distance from the shore of Lake Erie in Ohio to Chester, West Virginia (across the river from East Liverpool, Ohio), to be 103 miles.

The next question: How many miles to run each day? Or, looking at it a different way, how many days to spend in Ohio? I kicked around two approaches: five days with a 20.6-mile daily average or six days with a 17.1 average.

Making judgment, I heard two voices: Elaine's saying, "This is a vacation," and my 80-year-old body saying, "Let's not get carried away." Easy decision: six days at a 17.1 miles daily. (In actuality the distance turned out to be 102.5 miles and my daily average was 17.08 miles.)

Starting at Ohio's north border on the shores of Lake Erie, near Harbour Marina in Conneaut, I swung onto Park Avenue and from there on Mill Street, which in a mile or so connected with Highway 7 south. I stayed on 7 for the rest of the 15.0-mile day finishing a half-mile south of its junction with Highway 167.

Near the shores of Lake Erie the two-star attractions were the upscale Harbor View Condos and the long-established Hieckersels Family Restaurant. Going through Conneaut, I was taken with the beauty of the restored old homes along Mill Street and with the crafts-manship of the Amish carpenters.

From this loftiness I transcended to noticing, this being garbage day, that all the garbage was placed on the sidewalks in plastic bags – no garbage cans being used. Now that was something I'd never seen before.

As I went past St. Francis Xavier Cabrini church and school, my reaction was, Something else I've never seen before; didn't know there was a saint by that name.

Otherwise I saw nothing of particular note in Conneaut as I ran from Lake Erie to Highway 7. Nor did we see anything impressive yesterday in our drive around this city of 13,000 inhabitants. From what we saw, we deduced Conneaut's economy relies heavily on tourism.

After I crossed State Street and got onto Highway 7 the going was comfortable because I had the security of a bike lane. But also uncom-fortable because I was doing a lot of asthmatic hacking and in that I was running in rain.

Probably because he took pity on me in the rain, a good Samaritan stopped to offer a ride. "Thanks, but no thanks" was my response as I waved him on.

Elaine, probably trying to buoy up my morale in the rainy weather, made her first pit stop beside a supermarket and treated me to a couple of gooey donuts. So refueled, I hit the road in better spirits.

At the second pit stop I found Elaine still recovering from an experience with an Ohio Highway Patrol officer. With red lights flashing, he had pulled up behind her when she was parked for the pit stop. She hurried out to explain what we were doing.

"Oh, I wasn't citing you," he said, "just checking on what you were doing."

He asked Elaine to explain her sign in the back window of the motorhome that read, "No problem. Runner pit crew."

"That sign's a good idea," he said. "It saves questions. What you're doing is all right as long as you park outside the fog line."

Once I emerged from the Conneaut environs, the setting for the rest of the day was agriculture and farms. One noticeable feature of many of the farms was the oversized barns, about as big as a gymnasium.

From my roadside view the farming did not seem as well organized or operated as some in other states. The Meadowbrook Farm – with huge barns, many silos, all facilities and grounds well-kept – was an exception. It seemed that about every mile or so an old farm house, now abandoned, lay crumpling.

I was appalled at the condition of an old cemetery, about five miles into my day. Overgrown with grass and weeds, and with tombstones all askew, it looked like the aftermath of a hurricane. I did a quick check of tombstones and found one dating back to 1838 and many from the mid-1850s.

A short while later I came into Monroe Corner – consisting of residences, a town hall, no businesses and a United Methodist Church. Now there's an idea, I told myself: Methodists, why not take a Sunday off from church and devote your time and effort to straightening up that nearby cemetery?

When I first saw it coming toward me, I couldn't figure out what it was. As it got closer, I saw it was an Amish wagon. Since the wagon's wheels were on the fog line, I moved over to the other side of the road to give it room. I waved as the man and wife, both bundled in blankets, went past and they waved back.

By the time I had reached 15 miles, the rain had increased to a torrential tempo. I surrendered for the day, and we drove back to the Evergreen Lake Campground near I-90.

Normally this spacious facility under pine trees would have been a comfortable setting. But by the time we were hooking up amid thunder, lightning and torrential rain, the entire site was wet and muddy.

Actually, though, despite the rain, this first day in Ohio was somewhat easy, mainly because I had the protection of a bike lane, moderate traffic and some disassociating in adjusting to Ohio.

DAY TWO. What a glorious feeling this morning to run and not be hacking, coughing or gasping for air. Sort of a moratorium on asthma for some unknown reason.

Shortly after starting, I welcomed a change from the agricultural setting when I passed through Pierpont, a small town extending about a half-mile along Highway 7. Besides residences, Pierpont contained an elementary school, Masonic temple, garage, Citgo gas station, restaurant, hardware store and Andover Bank. Hardly exciting but at least a change from fields and farms.

After leaving Pierpont, I had a brief conversation with a farmer. He told me that his two main crops are corn and oats.

"I'm having a lot of trouble this year because of the weather," he said. "All the farmers around here are having the same trouble. It's a mess, things don't look good."

Both ends of the spectrum, I told myself, after passing two places – one positive, one negative. On the positive side a tidy, well-kept, prosperous looking farm with three huge barns, two silos and a two-story frame home of at least five bedrooms. On the negative side, down the road a bit a place that contained a couple of deteriorating sheds, three dilapidated cars, three motorhomes rusting away and a flagpole flying a Confederate flag.

Also on the premises were two dog houses atop of which stood dogs howling as I passed by. Will some dog psychologist explain why these dogs like to stand on top of their dog houses?

After going by a number of farms, I was beginning to suspect that the cattle here are on tranquilizers. Unlike the cattle in western states that stampede on seeing me, these simply stand and stare.

At an early pit stop Elaine reported on listening to the truckers on their CB radios. She heard them referring to "the old lady on the road with the radio." When their detailed descriptions told about a safari running cap, dark glasses, running shorts and a yellow T-shirt, she realized they were talking about *me*.

This is an all-time low, I told myself, but I've got to rise above it with humor. Sure, sure, musta been those sexy legs of mine that caused the truckers to think of me as an "old lady."

Reference to sexy legs swung me to thinking about my friend Stuart Honse. He had read an article in which some woman reporter had referred to my "sexy legs," and that caused him to fire off a letter to me "to set the record straight."

His letter described my legs in the most uncomplimentary terms – something like "bony chicken legs, bow-legged and with knobby knees." Stuart, my friend, you should have been listening to these truckers!

In his book, *The Ultimate Athlete*, George Leonard says, "Old men run as if they fear to leave the ground." For much of today I seemed to fit that mold.

A couple of observations as I went down the road. When I passed an Amish settlement and looked into a garage and expected to see a car, and instead saw an Amish wagon, the sight turned back the clock for me – back to a time preceding Henry Ford and the Model T.

Another observation: All the folks we've encountered so far in Ohio have been friendly. I'd guess that about 90 percent of the drivers move over for me. For her part Elaine says the residents have been understanding when she's asked to park in a driveway for a pit stop.

About 25 miles into Ohio I started to become aware that the route was much more difficult than I had anticipated. The biggest problem was that for many miles the two-lane highway had a drainage ditch on both sides of it and the top of the ditch came right to the edge of the road.

When the slope of the ditch permitted, I could stand at an angle on it when cars approached. Often, though, the ditch was an abrupt drop and no place for me to stand.

In such areas I had to stand in the home driveways that extended over the ditch. Often I was sprinting from driveway to driveway, and always I was making an estimate of whether I could reach a particular driveway before an approaching car descended on me.

I spaced out to some disassociating, making the miles go faster, when I remembered being perturbed when I recalled a recent "60 Minutes" show in which Ed Bradley reported a case of racial discrimination. My problem with Bradley's approach, as with so many other reporters, was that in their thinking discrimination is always and solely a case of whites picking on blacks.

Listen, Ed, let me tell you about something that happened to me.

Nothing to do with race, just to show you there are other kinds of discrimination.

In late December 1942, with United States in a state of war and three weeks prior to my shipping out, I was in Reno, Nevada, with family and friends. We decided to have a drink in the bar of the El Cortez Hotel.

As we were about to enter the bar, we saw a sign: "Military personnel in uniform not allowed." That included me, a first lieutenant in a Marine Corps uniform. Never mind that the USA had been at war for almost a year, never mind that I would soon be on a battlefield being shot at, never mind that once we were at war military and naval personnel were ordered to wear uniforms and no civilian clothing.

I never saw a "60 Minutes" special on that kind of discrimination, Ed. In fact, to widen the scope, never saw a "60 Minutes" special on the widespread discrimination that existed in America prior to World War II against enlisted military personnel.

What's that, Ed, you say you're concerned only with racial discrimination? Well, once I was on the receiving end of a minor bit of racial discrimination.

When the Marine Corps transferred me from Hawaii to the Mainland, my family and I returned home on a ship. We were housed in two small rooms, one with three bunks, the other with two bunk beds, and the toilets and showers were down the hall. At the same time a black Navy officer, much junior to me, and his family were assigned a large outside stateroom with beds, showers, toilets, best the ship had to offer.

Learning this, I asked the ship's officer who made room assignments, "I don't understand why a junior officer was assigned better quarters than I. Is the reason that he is a Navy officer and I'm a Marine, or what is the reason?"

"Oh," he replied, "it was not a Navy-Marine thing. We were afraid we might get accused of discrimination if a black officer did not get a good stateroom."

"You mean regardless of rank?" I asked.

"Yeah, something like that."

Know what, Ed, if the scenario were reversed, the black officer being the senior person with inferior assignment, I have the feeling you'd probably do a special on it.

Just as I had that thought, I was brought back to the road and reality when a Ford pickup stopped alongside me and I expected to see a male driver. Instead I heard Sandy Dale, a lady kind enough to ask, "Are you tired? Do you need a ride?"

As she drove off after I thanked her, again my thoughts harkened back to Stuart Honse. I wanted to tell him, "You see, Stuart, those darn sexy legs of mine just got me more attention!"

By 16.4 miles I was tired– primarily because the stormy weather kept us awake much of last night – so I quit and we headed for Pymatuning State Park for the night. The experience there gave us a bad opinion of the Ohio state park system.

We found out that there was no water or sewage hookup for motorhomes, and that in the entire camp there was only one faucet for filling the motorhome water tank.

While the park advertised electrical hookups, it had only 20-amp connections, not the 30-amp required to operate the motorhome air conditioner. They treated the people with dogs like lepers, confining them to one small area – the least desirable area of the park.

We had to fill out a complete registration form for each dog, something never required anyplace before. The form covered pedigree, rabies shots, vaccinations, license number and such. The registration for the dogs was much longer than the ones we had to fill out for ourselves.

The space we were assigned was nothing more than a parking spot on an open grassy field. In the past we had more inconveniences in other parks, but never before had we encountered such an attitude that said, You should realize that we're doing you a big favor by letting you and your dogs stay here.

The experience was enough to vow that we'd never again stay in an Ohio state park.

DAY THREE. "Very strange weather for this time of year," the natives told us. "It's usually 30 or 40 degrees hotter." Which is what I found myself wishing, 30 degrees hotter, as I started this morning with the temperature in the high 30s.

I was on the road but a short while when it became apparent that today, like yesterday, I'd have to contend with the same road problem: the drainage ditch with its abrupt drop-off beside the road.

Another problem was that the two-lane road had an average of less than two feet of pavement beyond the fog line and beyond the pavement a couple of feet of grass. Often I was stepping into grass not knowing what lurked there.

These two conditions, drainage ditch and no running shoulder, typify what often makes running across a state difficult. Most people, when talking to me about my running across states think only in terms of thousands and thousands of steps, just smooth running across a runnable pathway. Were it so, running across a state would then be a piece of cake.

But it doesn't work that way. What makes such running difficult is the struggle to find running space, the never-ceasing alertness to keep from getting whacked by an approaching vehicle.

Also adding to my woes and boo-hoo's today was a heavy increase in traffic, attributable by my guess to the upcoming Memorial Day holiday. An inordinate number of motorhomes, motorcycles and towed boats were on the road.

And in one area on Highway 7, between the junctions of Highways 82 and 62, I had to contend with a parade of semis, all bumper to bumper. I was told that by following this part of Highway 7 they could avoid scales somewhere in the area.

As with my previous Ohio days the setting was mostly the same, farms and agriculture. The most distinctive sign I saw of farmer prosperity was when I passed a three-story brick mansion with a three-car garage and adjacent airplane landing strip. Dollars dangling in all directions.

The towns of Hubbard and Brookfield provided some variety from the agricultural scenery. Hubbard set me off in several directions:

- "Paul's Place," what a crummy looking bar.
- "Macaroni Lodge," cheez, what a strange name. Whoops, correction: It's "*Marconi* Lodge," dating back to 1938.
- Well, look there, every one of those 21 (yes, I actually counted them) windows in the Kelley/Robb Funeral Home has an electrical candle light in it. These electric lights, shaped in size and glow to resemble candles, were lighted even in daylight, in many Ohio homes.

In Hubbard I also admired the outstanding design of St.Patrick's Church, full-length stained glass windows and a statue of the old snake charmer himself in front of the church.

Brookfield typified many small towns in that the most prominent building in town was a funeral home, in this case the Madasz Funeral Home, a three-story white frame building of splendid appearance. Beyond that about all I noticed in Brookfield was residences.

A number of manufacturing plants were spread along my route in the Hubbard-Brookfield area. Usually I was not able to identify what they made. Seeing a forklift driver in front of one, I asked, "What do you make here?"

His answer: "Just a lot of noise."

My reply: "Not a very marketable product."

"No, really," he said, waxing serious, "we make a polish."

I was not sufficiently curious to ask what kind, and besides if I did he might answer something like, "A wet one." He was sort of a contradiction: a big, burly, bearded guy sucking on a lollipop. Honest!

Running today was an effort for two reasons. First, the weather remained cold all day and I ran bundled in a Goretex running suit, which itself made the running difficult. Here I was succumbing to another affliction of old age: Cold weather is hard to tolerate.

A second difficulty: After I'd been on the road for about five miles, my asthma began acting up. Contending with asthma so many years, I've learned some basic lessons about it. For one thing, medical science has no cure. Secondly, with age it gets worse – more susceptibility, more severe attacks.

The trick with treatment is to keep the asthma abated as much as possible and to slow the worsening process, all the while remembering that asthma will be with me the rest of my life. The choice is to live with it, live around it, the best I can.

Things not too lively on the road, this was another of those days when I did considerable day-dreaming. In one part of this disassociating my memory went back more than 50 years when the lyrics of a song came floating back to me.

An odd song it was, one I'd never heard until on Guadalcanal when I listened to a guy named Donovan sing it a hundred times or more as he moved about our camp. Donovan was kind of a wild man. Among his eccentricities he carried a walking stick wherever he went.

And for some strange reason he impulsively broke out with this song several times a day. The frequency seemed to double when he was chosen to go into Bougainville.

Maybe the increased singing was because he was nervous. He had reason to be.

He went into the island three days before any Marines landed there. His mission was to observe and report any Japanese troop movements and to direct naval gunfire on the beach just prior to the landing. His only companion was his walking stick.

As for the song it could have been the only one in Donovan's repertoire. I never heard him sing anything else. So many times did I hear him sing it that, as I reminisced, I had no difficulty recalling the words. They went like this:

> *You can easily see she's not my mother*
> *Because my mother is 49.*
> *You can easily see she's not my sister*
> *Because I never showed my sister such a wonderful time.*
> *And you can easily see that she's not my sweetheart*
> *Because my sweetheart is too refined.*
> *She's just the kind of a kid*
> *Yes, the kind of a kid*
> *Who never cared what she did.*
> *She's just a personal friend of mine.*

Wacky song, and if I ever hear Donovan sing those words again, it will be in heaven. He was one of my Marine friends who never came back from the war.

Kind of odd, I thought, how I can recall the words of that song but can't for the life of me recall Donovan's first name. Strange, too, how Donovan should come to mind. Hadn't thought about the guy for ages, and such are the fallouts from being afoot on the road.

A few more observations as I plodded down the road today:

- The name Vindicator, which I saw on many newspaper delivery boxes, seemed oddball for a newspaper.
- In one area I could identify white pine and blue spruce trees because some botanist coached me with a sign describing them.
- What was uncommon about an apple orchard was that it was the first one I recall seeing this year.

- Unlike most small towns I've passed through, there were no historical markers in the towns on my route, or at least I have not seen any.
- Having been at dozens of races where dozens of portable potties are imported, I was impressed when I saw a customized trailer built to accommodate 10 toilets. So impressed that I photographed it and noted it was made by Leland Co., 501 S. Mill Dr., Pidgeon, MI 49099. Never can tell when a guy just might need one of these!

Our anticipated day's excitement was picking up some mail, forwarded by my daughter Nancy, to Hubbard. And it did turn out to be exciting for Elaine who received a summons to report for jury duty May 20th – that being yesterday.

At the end of our 16.1-mile day we overnighted at Chestnut Ridge RV Park, which turned out to be a delightful experience compared to the previous night at an Ohio state park.

DAY FOUR. Our route today was about equally divided between towns and agriculture as a setting. Not a single town offered any spectacular sight, but each did leave an impression or two.

In Struthers, for example, the most prominent building was not a funeral home as often seen in a small town, but instead a Catholic church with expansive landscaped grounds that held my attention to the point that I failed to get the name of the church. Struthers also contained the best homes – $300,000 to $400,000 range by California standards – I had seen since leaving Conneaut.

Of all things it was a barn, one of the European Swiss type, that caught my attention in Middleton. Still sturdy it stood after so many years of service. In different words there was nothing to see in Middleton.

In Petersburg I lingered a bit to admire four homes – all more than 100 year old, all well-preserved, all very livable. Such vintage made me feel like a kid.

More than once today I fell to wondering if the route across Ohio that Lou Abney had suggested would have been easier, more interesting – albeit I knew it was a bit longer. What made today's route tolerable and tenable was the consideration of the Ohio drivers and, except for the presence of some semis, the relatively light traffic.

However, two types of drivers in this state were inconsiderate: those driving sports vans and those driving local delivery trucks of three tons or under. But that was not unusual because those two types of drivers have been inconsiderate wherever encountered.

Oh, come to think of it, add school bus drivers to that list. Elaine had three instances in which they tailgated her even though she was at the legal speed limit, and every single school bus that approached me ran me off onto the shoulder.

If somebody were to ask, "What was the most impressive sight you saw in Ohio?" I'd unhesitatingly reply, "The 50 or more century or older homes I saw at various places along the way."

Each had a sign indicating its vintage. Each wore its age with charmed dignity. Everything about each place was absolutely immaculate.

By my recollection 90 percent of these homes were of wood frame, and the remaining 10 percent were brick. No two were alike.

As usual when on the road, I was looking around all the time, observing what I could. Some of the sights I took note of were these:

- By now I seem to have gone by an undue number of cemeteries in Ohio, and I have yet to see one that is properly maintained. At least 30 percent of the tombstones I saw today were askew.
- Here, similar to what I saw in western Pennsylvania, many homes posted signs reading "Go Tribe." No doubt about it, fans of the Cleveland Indians baseball team are abundant in these parts.
- The crop I saw most often was corn.
- All the residences along today's route had one thing in common: well-kept lawns.
- Seeing the concentration of residences in the various settlements – Struthers, Poland, New Middleton, Petersburg, East Palestine – along the way today left me wondering: Where do all these people earn a living? Is nearby Youngstown the answer?

My usual amount of reflecting on the road today did not mirror any dominant, lingering impression, such as my remembering of Donovan yesterday. Instead a hodge-podge of unrelated thoughts tumbled in my mind.

I recalled a marathon I'd run more than 20 years ago, one in which I did something entirely irrational and to this day I still don't know why. Part of the race course crossed the Golden Gate Bridge, north to south, at about the 23-mile mark of the race.

When I came to the north edge of the bridge, instead of going across the bridge I inexplicably ran down a dirt road, into Fort Baker and to the water's edge to the San Francisco Bay, a distance of at least a half-mile. Arriving at the water's edge, I suddenly realized my mistake and doing so was torn between cussing and crying.

In desperation, I even gave a fleeting and wild thought to swimming across the bay. Crushed and thoroughly pissed, I thought, You've come too far to quit. Then, steaming with anger, I ran back up the long hill, across the bridge and finished the marathon in 2:56.

I once logged a 2:39, but I suspect this one was faster. I don't suspect, I *know*, that the 2:39 was run much smarter.

I also thought about a remark often attributed to John F. Kennedy: "Life is not fair." Something I applied today to a couple of runners, Steve Scott and John Walker.

Scott has run 136 sub-four-minute miles; Walker, 124 of them. At one time not too long ago, precisely prior to Roger Bannister, a sub-four mile was considered humanly impossible.

Now where life is unfair is that for all their superb athleticism these two guys have been enriched miserly compared to the fabulous salaries of professional football, basketball and baseball players. What's the answer here: Is running too tame, without sufficient violence, for the American public?

Our day ended at 16.6 miles. Because we liked the Chestnut Ridge RV park in Hubbard so much last night, we drove 32 miles to overnight there again.

DAY FIVE. One of our plans in Ohio was avoiding going through metropolitan Youngstown if we possibly could. After studying our array of maps, we decided we could skirt the eastern edge of this city, coming within five miles of the metropolitan area.

This called for departing Highway 7 at its junction with I-80, near Hubbard, and finding and following Highway 616 south to the Struthers area where we would then seek out Struthers Road and take it south to the junction of Highway 170. From there we would take 170 south, which at one point near Petersburg came very close to the Pennsylvania border, about two miles by my quick estimate.

On the map this navigation looked simple. Reality, however, was a different matter because finding our way was often difficult. The road markings in some cases were not as we expected them, or they were nonexistent problems we wrestled with all the way after leaving the Hubbard area until we reached Highway 170.

In other words for a couple of days in Ohio we were not on the exact roads we wanted to be on. But we were always headed in the right direction, that being south.

Today we had special reason to be thankful for not taking Highway 7 through Youngstown. After finishing yesterday, we decided to drive 7 through Youngstown on our way to the Chestnut Ridge RV Park. The traffic was a nightmare.

Many of the roadways in Mahoning County, and even in Youngstown itself, were maintained about as badly as any we've seen. And to describe it kindly, Highway 7 passed through one very rough looking section of Youngstown.

As San Francisco 49ers football fans driving through Youngstown, we realized we were in the arena of the DeBartolo family, owners of the 49ers. By accident more than design, we drove past the Edward DeBartolo building, the family's business headquarters in Youngstown.

A disappointment. I would have expected more elegance, more class. I found the building devoid of class, of style.

This was another Ohio day with the problem of running some stretches of road with a drainage ditch and no shoulder. Another problem today was some rebellion from my asthma, which at times demanded attention. The good news was that I had no aches, pains or nagging injuries, which is a chorus many an 80-year old would like to sing.

Today, maybe as a fallout from some of our navigation problems, I found myself reflecting on some of the aspects of running across the country and states. I had to admit that before I every embarked on any of this, I was thinking only of footsteps – run, run, run.

More realistically, with time I have learned that the running, per se, is the easy part, the fun part. The land mines are the weather, careless drivers, inadequate running space, and the nuisance and demands of logistics.

Anything worthwhile involves time, effort and often sacrifices. Very true of our adventure. There were valleys and peaks all along the way.

I've come to learn to weather the valleys and to enjoy the peaks. I've been miserably hot, uncomfortably hot, dog-tired, scared in tornado warnings, but have never questioned, Is it worth it?

Just as combat – scary and stressful as it was – strengthened and improved me as a person, so have these running adventures. As in combat, once removed from the action, it is natural and easy to think back on all the running adventures as easier than they actually were.

People often ask me, "Isn't it boring being out there on the road all that time?" And my answer to that is, not at all.

In fact, one of the strongest forces that keeps me going on the road is the acrobatics that go on in my mind while I'm observing, reflecting, reminiscing, theorizing and just plain day-dreaming. One of the benefits of being out on the road is the luxury of thinking. I'm not bored when I go down the road because having my mind in gear is what makes it tenable and enjoyable.

I like all the meditative time. Going down the road absorbed in thought, I am sometimes oblivious to my running – something like making a long drive someplace, thinking all the way, arriving there and wondering how you ever got there.

At one point today I was so spaced out with my mental meandering that I ran right past Elaine, parked on a side street for a pit stop, without seeing her. I paid for that because, as a result, by the time she calculated that I'd missed her and then took off to catch up with me, I'd gone six miles without grub and grog.

Rough sledding for a softy spoiled with three-mile pit stops. Like Caesar said of Cassius, "He thinks too much; such men are dangerous."

Yes, being on the road is always exciting for me, never boring. Running has been good to me.

But there has been one negative fallout from it. That happens when I am personified or introduced as the runner – the inference often being that my world begins and ends with running, that jockville is the extent of my depth.

The most notable example of this happening to me was in a job interview conducted by a musical-chair superintendent (the type who lands a job in a school district and then immediately starts looking for upward mobility). He introduced me to the panel as "the runner" and, although he had no interest in the sport, devoted the first five minutes to talking about my running, a subtle put-down to typify me as a jock.

The irony here was that he himself had started his career as a high school baseball coach and that he graduated from a college to which I had a scholarship and refused it because the college ranked far below University of California, Berkeley, which I chose.

Now back to Ohio. Despite being in the state for five days, I still had not learned much about it. I already knew that the Ohio State football team had filled the 100,000-plus seats of its stadium for every home game for more than 30 years (whoops, that said, and I was just disclaiming jockville!).

I also knew that Ohio is called the "Buckeye State," and I even knew that seven presidents were born here. News to me, though, that George Armstrong Custer was born here – proving the old adage, You can't win em all!

The tidbit that I liked best about Ohio was that a guy named Harry M. Stevens, inspired by a cartoon of a dachshund, called the sandwich he introduced "a hot dog." Yes, take me out to the ball game!

The only interruptions from the agricultural and residential settings today were some charming century homes and a couple of towns along the way. East Palestine, the first city on today's route, billed itself as "A little city with a big future." Well, with a population of 5168 it had room for growth.

A real change of pace here in that the most attractive building in town was the public library, a new brick structure. The downtown area was buzzing with activity, but I didn't have the faintest idea of what was generating it.

In the town of Negley, with only 900 dwellers, both the residences and businesses seemed tired and worn out. The action in town seemed to revolve around the Volunteer Fire Department's bingo games on Tuesday nights.

All told, this was not a very lively day, but it did move us down the road another 16.7 miles.

DAY SIX. The bells were ringing, the birds were singing this morning because, for the first time in Ohio the weather was kind – the temperature comfortable enough for me to be running in T-shirt and shorts. Besides, the morale flag fluttered high because I knew that a little over 21 miles today would get us through Ohio.

Unlike most state routes so far this year, our Ohio route was devoid of historical markers. So seeing one today just north of Fredricktown was somewhat of a surprise. The marker read:

"The Great Trail of colonial times crossed the ridge at this point... Here stood the Rising Sun Tavern, an early stagecoach hostelry on the Pancake/Carson Road. Also called the Tuscarawas Trail."

Nearby was a nursery owned by Pancake and Sons. Pardon me, sir, but I do have a hard time holding a straight face when saying, "Mr. Pancake."

Elaine had an experience early in the day that got to her. This was meeting a high school boy who was taking care of his grandparents.

She was parked in front of their home and the boy came out to talk with her. She learned that the grandmother had Alzheimer's, and that the grandfather depended on an oxygen hookup for his breathing and on a walker for his mobility.

When Elaine explained what we were doing, the boy, Brian, expressed considerable interest. The upshot of it was that Elaine gave him a copy of *Ten Million Steps*. Good move, the least we could do for a kid so devoted to his grandparents.

In Fredricktown I stopped for a brief chat with Gary Winterbann and Charles Stearns, two constables from Beaver Kennel Farms. They said that the 5000 acres of privately owned land they patrol is the largest such tract of land in Ohio.

Eighteen miles of Beaver Creek, a national scenic river, flow through it. The tract is a wilderness area with much wildlife, but the owners have homes on it. Starting the uphill climb out of Fredricktown and crossing Beaver Creek, I got a first hand look at the fast flowing stream, about 60 feet across.

The climb out of Fredricktown, about a nine-percent gradient, was the toughest hill I negotiated on our way across Ohio.

Calcutta, another town on our route, was so small (gas station, convenience store, pizza) that it offered nothing memorable, though I would have liked to sample Bruno's pizza. Considering the town's population is only 1212, the local folks must have a fixation on pizza to keep Bruno in business.

Several times today I thought back on a conversation which Elaine and I had last night about heaven. I couldn't remember how it got started, but I did remember we started with the assumption that heaven exists, contrary to the thinking of Russell Francis Burton who wrote, "There is no heaven, there is no hell. These are the dreams of baby minds."

I couldn't buy Elaine's basic tenet: that if a person believes in Christ and sincerely asks Him to forgive their sins, that person is ticketed for heaven. And she couldn't buy my thinking that heaven is not a free ride but rather something earned by adhering to certain moral precepts.

My key word here is "earned." Her key word is "belief."

Another point she was strong on is that people assume recognizable forms in heaven and are reunited with family and friends. While I did not question that at one time, I do now.

For one thing, granted that heaven is a place of perfect happiness – and there should be no argument with that – how can a person be perfectly happy with an earthly body that had many imperfections? Another consideration, say a person has been married twice or more; how are relationships worked out in heaven so that everyone is perfectly happy?

Then there's the matter of being in heaven with family and friends, and her contention that they are all aware of every bad deed you did, every bad thought you've had. Can you be perfectly happy knowing that? I'm not very comfortable with that idea.

St. Paul reported having a vision of heaven. If that were so, for a man of his intelligence and writing ability he was of no help in telling us about it. His words were something to the effect of, "The eye has not seen, the ear has not heard."

I don't know what the eye will see, but hopefully it will be more than a beehive of angels flapping their wings, and hopefully the ear will hear more than harps. Though both are the usual depiction of heaven.

The only thing I know for sure about heaven and hell is words I remember from *Paradise Lost* that go, best as I can remember: The mind can make a hell out of heaven and a heaven out of hell. And so can some psychiatrists!

From thinking about heaven, I switched to prostate cancer. The momentary terror when Dr. Erby Satter told me, "I'm sorry, Paul, but it's malignant."

My immediate reaction: What can I do about it? Telling Elaine, her instant resolve that the two of us would beat it.

Then, after the diagnosis, we weighed the decisions: a prostatectomy, radiation, do nothing (and live five years, I was told)? We chose 36 radiation treatments, 6400 rads, with Elaine insisting on driving me to the oncology facility every early morning, then sharing breakfast treats afterward.

I fulfilled my resolve to jog five miles on each of the 36 days of radiation, something I did more to boost my morale than for any other reason. Gradual recovery followed, working to return to normalcy. Then came the joy of returning to racing (a 10-K) within seven weeks after the radiation.

In subsequent years of monitoring, of PSA tests, I've puzzled over what I would do if the cancer flared up again. And, yes, I've questioned if radiation was the right choice – something I couldn't help thinking after such luminaries as Bob Dole, Arnold Palmer and General Norman Schwartzkopf all elected a prostatectomy.

But overriding everything else is the gratitude that my cancer has not metastasized, the appreciation for being able to continue active and the renewed joy of life. Yes, the trip down prostate gulch had its good points.

From the running perspective Ohio was difficult for me, mainly because my asthma acted up every day there. Sometime between two and four A.M. I'd awaken with an asthma attack (most books euphemistically call them "asthma episodes") and, choking and coughing, gasp for air for anywhere from 30 to 60 minutes. Between gasps I would try to sip some coffee or spray with an inhalant for relief.

On the road around eight A.M. I was still coughing and hacking, trying to expel phlegm. After a couple hours on the road I usually settled down to just labored breathing.

As I went along, I found myself not tired but disappointed that I was not running faster because my asthma kept me from sustaining a long, steady run. I had to stop every so often to walk a few steps and adjust my breathing.

On the positive side I marveled at how my feet, knees and legs were holding out so well. No complaints whatsoever.

Nearing the end of my day, I went past an elementary school that gave me cause to think about Maureen Meyer, a teacher at Wilmer Loomis Elementary School in Broomall, Pennsylvania. She had read portions of our book *Ten Million Steps* to her fourth-grade class and seemingly interested the kids in our adventure.

Each student had written to Elaine and me, most of them asking questions. Elaine and I got a kick out of some of the questions, and we answered each letter.

They requested pictures, which we sent. In return each kid sent us a picture and we received school T-shirts signed by each student. The experience was uplifting.

The biggest change in our scenery today was the transit through East Liverpool. With a 13,654 population it was cosmopolitan compared to what we had been seeing, Youngstown excluded.

I had some concerns about approaching East Liverpool on Highway 7, which south of Calcutta was a divided freeway. Luckily we discovered Highway 447 that pretty much paralleled it and went into downtown East Liverpool.

Much of 447 was a downhill slope, so the running was easy. The problem here was that a while before I reached 447, the Ohio weather turned on us and we were in a heavy rainfall and committed to continuing if we wanted to finish the state this day. Since the road sloped downhill and the rain was so heavy, I was running a creek as the rain flooded the road.

The inadequate drainage was one of the first things I noticed about East Liverpool. The streets were flooded. Also many of the city's sidewalks were torn up

The general impression of East Liverpool was that it was a beaten, battered city, many old buildings, and generally in considerable need of revitalization. The mood was depressing.

My intent as I meandered through the streets of the city was to cross the bridge over the Ohio River and to finish in Chester, West Virginia. That plan was sabotaged when I learned that pedestrians were not allowed on the bridge.

In the East Liverpool area the Ohio River forms the southern boundary of Ohio. Technically, to get to the Ohio/West Virginia border I should have been mid-river. But the best I could do was to find an overpass over Highway 30/11 that parallels the river, cross the overpass, then get onto a road leading to the west bank of the river.

Standing at the water's edge, I had no urge to swim halfway across the river to be in West Virginia. Besides, I was already drenched enough from the rain.

Because of the weather we lingered only a few minutes at the water's edge, and after taking a studied look at the bridge and Chester, West Virginia, across the water, we got in the motorhome and headed for our next state. We drove to Newell and, guess what, we spent the night at an RV park on the west bank of the Ohio River.

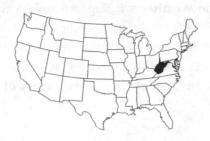

Chapter 9

West Virginia

Along the Historic National Road

Date: *May 25th, 1997*
Miles: *15.4*
Route: *Start at Pennsylvania/West Virginia border on Highway 40
and follow 40 west to Wheeling and bridge over Ohio River to Ohio
border.*

I had a heap of reasons for wanting to follow Highway 40 on my
run across West Virginia. The reasons lined up like this:

1. I would be treading on history since Highway 40 hereabouts
traced the historic National Road.
2. I reasoned that these days Highway 40 in this area should be
lightly traveled since it has been superseded by I-70.
3. Transferred from coast to coast on Marine Corps tours of duty,
I'd driven much of 40 and had last seen this area around 1954.
I was anxious to revisit.
4. I wanted another look at historic Wheeling, the fifth-largest city
in the state, despite having a population of only 35,000.
5. Compellingly the panhandle route across West Virginia (on I-70
or Highway 40) was the shortest distance across the state.

As my run unfolded, I found little along the way to memorialize
the National Road. From a couple of plaques I was reminded that it
originated in Cumberland, Maryland (for which reason it was also
known as the "Cumberland Road"), in 1811, and when construction
ended in 1852, it extended 800 miles to Vandalia, Illinois.

Seeing along the route some old cement mile markers, giving the distance to Wheeling, I deduced they were hangovers from the National Road. Definitely a hangover were some of the stopping houses that sprang up to serve traffic on the route. I took note of one, the Heimberger House, that had weathered the years gracefully.

I guessed correctly about Highway 40 being lightly traveled–at least until I reached the southern outskirts of Wheeling. As for revisiting an area of Highway 40 over which I had made previous trips, I failed to see one familiar sight. It was all news to me; couldn't recall any scene or setting along the way.

Even Wheeling unfolded without a trace of familiarity. I didn't even recall the city's famous 900-foot suspension bridge–one of the world's longest, dating back to 1849 and providing passage over the Ohio River. (Original tolls for this passage were 10 cents for a man and horse, 15 cents for a six-horse carriage and two cents each for hogs and sheep.) Nor did I recall how picturesquely Wheeling sits on the banks of the Ohio River.

I was right on target, though, about Highway 40 being a short route across this state. From the West Virginia/Pennsylvania border on 40 to the Ohio River, the distance I ran was a mere 15.4 miles.

Even though I was running in the "Mountain State," almost all my route was flat. The exceptions were a hilly area near the start and some hills on the outskirts of Wheeling before the road descended into the city.

Wheeling was the only city of size on my route, but I did go through a couple of other communities. The first was Valley Grove, a small town spread out over a mile in four different clusters in a narrow pass.

The community included a volunteer fire department, a motel with no vacancies (even the honeymoon suite was occupied!), Assembly of God Church, small variety store, an attractive city park with a basketball court and picnic area. All this excitement happened shortly after I got underway.

The other community was Triadelphia, about halfway into my running day. Spread out over 1.5 miles, it consisted of modest homes on both sides of the road, a garage, bar and grill, a cabinet shop, small coffee shop and two churches (Methodist and Catholic with the unusual name of Our Lady of the Seven Dolors). In the entire community only one building, a two-story framed apartment house, had any semblance of being modern.

What intrigued me about Triadelphia was a plaque telling how it got its name. It said the town was named for three friends and went on to describe them as Jonathan Link, who built a block house near here in 1780, and his two companions, Wesley Peak and Tommy Hawkins, who were captured and killed by Indians. I'm still trying to figure out how Triadelphia evolved from Link-Peak-Hawkins.

Though West Virginia is noted for its scenic beauty, I saw nothing breath-taking along Highway 40. I did pay considerable attention, though, to a stream about 30 feet wide that paralleled our route.

Swollen by recent rains, it was a raging torrent – muddy, carrying much debris, threatening to crest its banks. In fact, in one spot the highway maintenance department was working frantically to control some overflow.

Here Elaine had to drive through water up to the hubcaps of the motorhome, water I was able to avoid by retreating to the high ground on the other side of the road. This stream crossed under the road at times, the most notable spot being at Elm Grove Stone Bridge, built in 1817 as part of the National Road. A plaque told me that the bridge was constructed of uncoursed limestone but was covered by concrete in 1958.

The route did have more than its share of historical plaques. Besides the one pertaining to the National Road, stopping places, Valley Grove, Triadelphia, there were some others.

One described Fort Henry, and from it I learned that the last battle of the Revolutionary War was fought here (actually after the cessation of hostilities). Another told about a guy named Gray, born in Valley Grove, who developed some arithmetic and algebra books that were widely used – and about which I'd never before heard.

But very vividly I can recall old Brother Mark teaching us arithmetic. If we didn't solve the problems fast enough to suit him, he might hasten the process by tapping us (none too gently) on the hands with his pointer stick. Another marker commemorated the West Virginia birthplace, organized in 1861 at Washington Hall, Wheeling.

Not enough that I was overwhelmed with plaques. There were also statues.

One called "Madonna of the Trails" was dedicated to all the pioneer mothers. Another was an eight-foot bronzed statue of an Indian with the inscription, "Mingo, the original inhabitants of this valley, extend greetings and peace to all wayfarers."

A couple of billboards along the way caught my attention. One advertised the 21st Big Boy 20-K Classic, Saturday, May 24th. I felt not even a trickle of temptation to stick around for this event.

The other billboard read, "Jody, please forgive me. I love you [followed by three hearts of art work]. Greg."

Leaving many of us – well, certainly me – to wonder what terrible thing did Greg do? Let's hope, was my thought, that if the deed were indeed dastardly, Jody is not swayed by this showmanship.

A joyous feeling this day to look overhead, see the cloudless sky and know that I'd finish this run without any rain. This was much appreciated after a couple of days of downpour in this area, as testified to by the raging stream paralleling the road.

A good feeling it was, too, to be running with no strain, no pain. Partly due, most probably, to the fact that I was moving at a slow, comfortable pace. Or maybe I was relaxed just because I knew I had such a short distance to cover today.

Another consideration was that I was doing most of my running on the cinder-gravel shoulder instead of on the road itself, saving the energy of jumping back and forth from road to shoulder. By no means was I a ball of fire. But, and I blush at mentioning this, for an 80-year old I felt like a hot dogger!

At times I found myself wishing this National Road could talk. What tales it could tell!

Once I reached the outskirts of Wheeling, there was more to see than I could take in. I was caught off guard by all the magnificent mansions that lined one section of the National Road.

Maybe I'd heard too many hillbilly songs, seen too many depictions of impoverished West Virginians to be prepared for this. These were three-story homes with manicured grounds and of varying types of architecture – stately homes that radiated more character than the mansions, say, of Bel Air.

In stark contrast were two other housing areas along the route. In one of these areas the homes on the north side of the road sat up from the road 30 or 40 feet on a flat section of the ridge.

The only access was by the steps from the road.

Directly across the street the entrance to the homes was at street level and from there down steps 30 or so feet to the homes that sat on a flat section of the ridge. The only access to the homes was on these steps.

In both cases, north and south, home owners had to park their cars on the street. I couldn't help but think of what gut-busting labor it had to have been to get the building materials to the sites of these homes.

I came upon the other housing on the eastern tip of downtown Wheeling. The road sloped downward here, and all the homes were situated directly adjacent to the sidewalk. It was but one step from the sidewalk to the front door, one step from the sidewalk to the home's windows. Small homes, old homes, devoid of any privacy.

I didn't get much of a feel for downtown Wheeling, mainly because it was a Sunday and there was no action downtown. Observing some of the buildings and stores, I saw more urbanity and sophistication than I had expected in Wheeling.

Once in the downtown area I was thankful it was Sunday because I had no traffic problems scooting down the sidewalk, arriving at the Highway 40 bridge and going out to the Ohio River which marked West Virginia's west boundary.

As my thoughts wandered this day, I found them at one point focused on World War II. In the heat of battle I was preoccupied exclusively with doing my job and surviving, though I did sometimes, when seeing comrades killed or wounded, reflect on how lucky I was escaping without even a wound.

But it was not until sometime months after the cessation of hostilities, when out of the war zone and now in a peaceful setting, that I came to recognize and understand that these war years were privileged time for me. For many reasons.

Never again would I experience as close a camaraderie as felt among comrades in arms. I never remember us speaking of this affection for each other, this willingness to risk our lives for each other, but we knew the feeling was there.

Never again, short of another war, would I be a player on such an important team, none better, and none for a more noble cause. The stakes, life and death, were so high that by comparison something like the Super Bowl ranked as kid stuff.

Never again would I be positioned to give so much for my country. Often, prior to combat, I had asked myself, Under fire how would I measure up? By the grace of God, I was not found wanting, though I was scared as hell at times.

Since war can be so horrible, so repugnant, I almost felt guilty at times that I enjoyed my combat job so much. I actually had a ball on D-day at Guam, Peleliu and Okinawa, doing my job.

While I did not realize it at the time, immersed in combat, I came to realize later that the war was a profoundly influencing and exciting experience in my life. It helped to mold me. Ironic as it may sound, I feel a bit sorry for those who have never experienced war.

Such sentiments may get me pegged as a war monger, or a wacko. But, what the hell, such was the way the thoughts flowed in West Virginia.

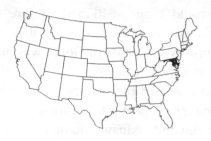

Chapter 10

Maryland

Pennsylvania to West Virginia via Cumberland

Date: *May 27th, 1997*
Miles: *7.1*
Route: *Start on Highway 220 at Pennsylvania/Maryland border and follow 220 south to Cumberland. Take Highway 28A south to cross Potomac River into Ridgely, West Virginia.*

After I thought about it for a while, where to run in Maryland was an easy choice. When I looked at the state map and saw that the Chesapeake Bay divided the state in two parts, I instantly decided that I'd run somewhere west of the bay.

Highway 219 – north-south from the Pennsylvania border to the West Virginia border, a distance of 50 miles or so – looked appealing. That is until John Wismer, a Maryland resident and Marine Corps classmate, sent me a newspaper article describing how black bears were overrunning this area.

"Lurid tales of bears killing horses and cornering hunters have grown with the animals return," the article reported. Enough to make me cease and desist on Highway 219. Elaine, animal lover that she is, would have preferred that I frolic with the bears.

Then in search of a short route across the state, I hit the jackpot. I learned that the narrowest width across any of the 50 states is in Maryland. It's only one mile across, from Pennsylvania to West Virginia, near Hancock, Maryland.

I already felt somewhat guilty about the short distances I'd run across some states. One mile was so short that the guilt would have driven me to confession. Jettison Hancock.

Up next popped Cumberland. Good Lord, why hadn't I thought of it before? Here's a place rich in American history: among other things, the east terminus of the National/Cumberland Road and the west terminus of the Chesapeake-Ohio Canal (never mind that by the time it was completed along came the Baltimore and Ohio Railroad to overpower it).

And the Maryland distance via Cumberland was cozy, too – only about eight miles by my reckoning, but legitimately across the state north-south from Pennsylvania to West Virginia.

As I started north of Cumberland on Highway 220, also called the "Pine Ridge Road," there were no landmarks. Only a sign told me I was at the Pennsylvania border.

The first half-mile was difficult and downright dangerous. There was absolutely no shoulder, and the semi traffic was heavy.

The curvy, downhill road had a guard rail on the edge of the fog line. When a vehicle approached, I had to jump the rail to get off the road. By the end of the half-mile I felt like a steeplechaser, and a pooped one at that.

Once past the guard rail I found the going easier. The road had a grass shoulder of about 14 inches and beyond that weeds into which I could flee.

Within the first couple of miles I was surprised to come into the community of Bedford because it was not shown on my maps. Bedford was a residential community of modest middle-class homes. The hilly forested ridge extended all the way to the back yards of these homes.

Going downhill shortly after leaving Bedford, I passed a young woman jogger, in her 30s by my guess. She was wearing a Walkman and listening intently to it.

I got within a foot or two of her before she realized I was there. Startled, she half-stumbled as I went past.

I had two reactions. My first was how foolhardy for a woman jogger to wear a Walkman, making it easy for anyone to sneak up on her; too many creeps in today's society for such exposure. My second reaction, more deep-seated, was how tragic that a jogger is missing one of the main benefits of distance running – that being the setting running provides for meditation and reflecting on life and for trying to solve problems. Invariably I find that my mind is more in gear, more active, when I am running than when I am stationary.

About all I saw the next three miles or so was houses – all uniformly modest, say lower-middle class and neat. The only exception was an occasional vintage home and some row homes.

Except for the hectic first half-mile, I ran relaxed all day, knowing I had slightly less than eight miles to do. Which brought to mind one of the big contrasts between the USA run and the subsequent state runs.

On USA there was always the drama of whether I'd make it – 3192 miles from coast to coast. Maybe I'd get sick, injured or plain frazzled and fatigued. Or Elaine, a vital link to my success, could get sick. Also there was always the possibility of the motorhome breaking down.

Contrastingly as I begin each of the state runs, there is little doubt that I'll get across.

Once I reached the outskirts and sidewalks of Cumberland, I was completely relaxed. Sidewalks meant I would no longer have to dodge cars and trucks.

History speaks, I thought, as I crossed Highway 40 that follows the same route here as did the National Road/Cumberland Road of the early 1800s – the same Highway 40 I had followed across West Virginia. As I crossed over the freeway, Interstate 68, I got a good look at the Cumberland skyline and decided I'd detour a bit, play tourist and see some of the downtown area.

Along the way I stopped to photograph two buildings: Bell Tower Building (the name comes from its being topped by a square wooden bell tower), dating from 1884 and first used as a police headquarters and jail and now housing the Chamber of Commerce. The second photo was of the Cumberland City Hall, dating from 1911, noted mainly for its marble interior and mural of General Edward Braddock and George Washington.

Downtown, jogging on the brick-lined pedestrian mall, I did draw a few strange looks. Taking in the downtown area, I concluded that Cumberland, for a city of its size (24,000) reflected sophistication.

I was brazen enough, in T shirt and shorts, to invade a bookstore to look at its selection of "local books." A tome on the National Road, priced at $35, looked appealing, but I had neither the money to buy it nor the energy to carry it.

A French bakery also caught my eye and left me drooling. We'll drive back here after I finish and get some goodies, I thought. Didn't materialize, though, because I couldn't sell the idea to Elaine.

I even made a detour to the West Maryland Station Center on Canal Street. My motive was to stop at the Visitor Center housed there, along with four other offices. There I talked with Pat Sweitzer of the Allegheny County Visitors Bureau, who imparted some information about the old National Road.

Among the things I remember her telling me was that President Jefferson signed legislation in 1806 creating the Cumberland Road, and this was the only road construction bill named after a town.

"There was a big delay, though," she said, "because the contract to build the first 10-mile section from Cumberland was not let until 1811."

She went on to say that once work started, there were all kinds of problems. The weather did not cooperate, the workers complained of low wages, stripping away the scrub growth and oak trees was difficult, mistakes in surveying were made by people who were not engineers, and building materials were stolen."

"Despite all the problems," she went on, "by 1816 the pike was completed from Cumberland to Uniontown at a cost of $9476 per mile, and it was considered to be the best-constructed road in America at the time."

I learned that upwards of a thousand freight wagons had made the trip in 1818 with loads averaging two tons, and subsequent years brought increased traffic. The road was subject to much depreciation, and Congress had to appropriate funds to repair it.

"You know," she continued, "most people think it was a toll road from its very beginning. That's not true. It did not become a toll road until 1835."

The tendency is to think of the road being used exclusively by wagons and stagecoaches, but that, too, is not true. Over it traveled horses from Texas, cattle from Illinois, mules and sheep from Ohio, and thousands of swine from Indiana and Ohio.

In fact, the swine did become a problem for the citizens of Cumberland. In 1839 they voted to outlaw pigs on the main thoroughfare.

Pat suggested that Elaine and I might want to ride the Western

Maryland Scenic Railroad, a steam train excursion lasting 3-1/2 hours and traveling from Cumberland to Frostburg. Good idea, I told her, but we could not do it because of our dogs.

Leaving the Visitor Center, I had a little trouble getting oriented and finding my way to Green Street, which lead to Ridgely and West Virginia.

At Riverside Park I came upon a building, first erected in 1755, that served as George Washington's headquarters during the French and Indian Wars. Later, when president, Washington used the building in 1794 to inspect troops of the Whiskey Rebellion.

I photographed the building and learned about it by playing the self-operated tape on the front porch. The building was restored in 1921.

The entire building did not appear to be bigger than 20 by 20 feet. Sort of cramped for a guy George's size, I thought.

Almost immediately after leaving Riverside Park, I crossed the Potomac River. More history. The Civil War song, "All Quiet Along the Potomac," came to mind.

Fifty yards down the road I found Elaine waiting for me. "Wherever have you been?" she asked.

I did not want to confess that, among other things, I had dallied at a bakery and bookstore. "Oh, I got a little lost in town and wandered around losing some time," I replied. An honest but somewhat evasive answer.

The total distance across Maryland turned out to be only 7.1 miles by Elaine's measure, which did not include my meandering around downtown Cumberland.

As we headed for lunch to celebrate Maryland, I tallied where we stood on our 1997 running schedule. The answer: 10 states completed, 11 yet to run in the East, then only Alaska and Hawaii and we'd be finished with all 50 states. Almost beginning to see the light at the end of the tunnel.

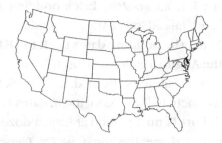

Chapter 11

Delaware

Washington Also Crossed It

Date: *May 29th, 1997*
Miles: *14.1*
Route: *Start at Delaware River, New Jersey/Delaware border, go through Port Penn and take County Road 2 west to Boyd's corner on Highway 13. Cross 13 and follow Boyd's Corner/Churchman Road to Maryland border.*

Knowing that Delaware is the second-smallest state in the country, I reasoned it would be easy to find a short route across the state. And that's just what John Harvison, a runner and native of Wilmington did for me. The distance was all of 14.1 miles.

John suggested that I start on the shores of the Delaware River at the municipal parking lot/boat ramp in the small town of Port Penn. John's route went west along Port Penn Road, Pole Bridge Road, crossed Highway 13 at Boyd's Corner Road, then followed Churchman Road to the Maryland border. Just to make sure I would not get lost, John even sent me a map of the route.

Walt Pierson, who is two-thirds through running the 330-mile length of the Delaware River, also made some helpful suggestions.

Where I started was in the area also known as Augustine Beach. I thought it might be named after St. Augustine. Instead, so I learned, it was named after Augustine Hermann, who mapped the Delaware Peninsula in the mid-1600s for Lord Calvert of Baltimore. Oh well, maybe Mr. Hermann was named after St. Augustine.

Across the street (this being Congress Street) from the start stood

Schmidt's Augustine Inn, a two-story brick building. To find out about it, I went inside and talked with the bartender, who was without customers. He told me the building dates back to 1814 and that it was originally called the Augustine Beach Hotel.

"The two adjacent buildings," he said, "date back to 1790." Seemed to make sense inasmuch as Port Penn, itself, dates back to 1763.

Going through Port Penn, I passed at least a dozen vintage homes. The one that impressed me the most was a Georgian-style house, brick, three stories. I stopped to photograph it and read about it. I found out it was called "Linden Hall," built in 1845. Its value then, when it was the town's finest house, was $2500.

I briefly admired the two churches that have graced the local landscape for more than a century: the Port Penn Presbyterian Church, founded in 1836 and rebuilt in 1856, and St. Daniel's United Methodist Episcopal Church dating from 1844.

The only business I saw in town was a combination cafe-convenience store. Without success I tried to purchase some post cards of the area.

My other stop in Port Penn was at Port Penn Interpretive Center. There I had a brief chat with Mary Smith, the curator, who explained that the exhibits are intended to represent Delaware's traditional cultural values and wildlife.

Among other things there was a mounted specimen of each of the varmints that have inhabited the area. I was glad to see no mountain lion.

Once out of Port Penn I found myself on a narrow, two-lane road without any shoulder for running. The saver was minimal traffic. Much of the area was under cultivation and, where it was not, homes or forestation dotted the landscape.

When I arrived at my first pit stop, Elaine asked, "What took you so long?" Whereupon I had to explain about my visits to the inn, the cafe, the Interpretive Center and photographing some buildings.

"Well," she replied, "all you needed to make your day complete was an old bookstore."

Down the road a short distance I encountered Maynard Rasch, a retired gent who was busy doing some serious fishing from a bridge.

"What kind of fish you fishing for?" I asked.

"Crappie, mainly," he said.

"That's a fish I never heard of," I admitted.

"Oh, they're pretty common around here," he said. "Most of them are about 10 to 12 inches long."

I took note of the muddy water and of the stream's name, Augustine Creek. At least this time I knew it was not named after St. Augustine.

Maynard went on to say, 'There are also catfish and white perch here. And once in a while I catch a bass if I am lucky."

Intent on his fishing, Maynard had not the slightest interest in what I was doing. Didn't he know I'm a sensitive soul!

As I went on, the scenery in this area was not very exciting – agriculture, some forestation and a few gullies. When the road dipped into a gully, I had to be especially careful because a car could suddenly descend on me without the driver seeing me or seeing me too late. A happenstance which could be fatal for me.

I did some disassociating along this stretch as I mulled what I had read last night in James Michener's book, *Quality of Life*. The first thing that surprised me about the book was that I had anticipated it would be focused on things personal, whereas the focus was on the nation.

For example, Michener talked about what he called the sources of America's strength, these being the Constitution, education, economy, abundance and religion. To me there seemed to be something missing in that equation.

The more I thought about it, the missing ingredient, at least to me, was the American people themselves. People who are by their nature imbued with unusual initiative and resourcefulness.

I remembered that after I read the chapter in which he detailed six areas of concern for the nation, I had to flip through it a second time to make sure I had not missed something. Michener listed the city, race, education, youth, communications and environment.

I kept looking for crime. It was nowhere to be found. To me crime (including the drug scene) would rank as the number-one concern in America. What was I missing here?

I had to applaud one thing Michener said: When he was teaching, he believed his first responsibility was to maintain order so that learning could take place. Bingo, he put his finger on the number-one problem in American education.

It's that simple. Yet much "educationalese" focuses on such things as class size, computers in the classroom and testing, without any regard for maintaining order in the classroom.

Absorbed in thought, I came to Highway 13 and immediately saw I faced a problem getting across this divided highway at Boyd's Corner where a number of roads converged. In fact, I counted 11 different stop lights.

The road was a virtual race track. As I studied it, I saw an area about a quarter-mile away where the traffic thinned and where I had a chance of crossing. I jogged there and eventually worked my way across the road.

Now on Churchman's Road I did a double-take when I went past Abrendbrum's Kennel and Cattery. What the hell is a cattery?

Must have something to do with cats, the best I could deduce. The John Madden type would be saying, what about a doggery?

The thought that hit me most when I saw a huge granary on Highway 301 was that I had underestimated the extent of agriculture in Delaware. Ever the curious one I stopped in at the granary and talked with Ray Woodward, the person in charge.

"This granary holds 885,000 bushels," Ray told me. I was amused to find myself thinking, Odd number. Why didn't they go for an even million?

When I told Ray about my route, he informed me I'd be passing the DuPont Farms with a number of race horses and also by the Taylor Farms, owned by a Canadian liquor distiller, also noted for its race horses.

"Both farms have produced champions," Ray told me.

In fact, I did not get a close view of either place. They were both fenced and gated, and trees obstructed the view. In the distance I could see stables and elaborate buildings. A series of corrals re-minded me of Kentucky, but despite all the elegance the grass was no match for Kentucky's.

In this area I didn't need a tour guide to tell me I was passing through affluence. By my estimate none of the homes there would sell for less than $400,000 in my part of California.

Moseying through horse country resurrected memories of times when horses played a role in my life. The first instance I could think of harkened back to my grammar school days when I spent summers at Richardson Springs, near Chico, California, where my mother worked.

Bobby Richardson, my age, had free access to some Shetland ponies the Springs owned. Quite understandable since his grandparents owned the Springs. One of our favorite pastimes was to saddle up a couple of ponies and play Pony Express.

During our role playing as Pony Express riders, Bobby insisted on being called "Buffalo Bill," and he persisted in calling me Pablo. I did not quite understand why until he explained that it meant "Paul" in Spanish. From the gutsy and game Shetlands I learned that good things can come in small packages.

My next exposure to horses was on my uncle's ranch. In my high school days I spent part of my summers there, and one chore I had was to assist him with his deer hunters. The horse I rode doing this was named Prince because, my uncle said, he looked so regal the first time he saw him.

By the time I came to ride him, Prince was in his declining years. But he was a gentleman, patiently tolerating my bumbling horsemanship.

The hunting procedure was that my uncle would start with his dogs on the open end of a horseshoe canyon and flush the deer out to the hunters, who were on strategic stands waiting to shoot the flushed out deer. My job was to lead the hunters to their stands. I had no difficulty locating the stands because Prince had been through the routine so many times he lead me to them.

Over the three summers I rode him, Prince and I developed a mutual affection. When I came back for a fourth summer, Prince was no longer living. Without him it was a lousy summer.

From thinking of Prince, I fumbled to think of the last time I rode a horse. Then it came to me: at Yellowstone when Elaine and I took grandkids, Joe and Cyndie, then 12 and 10, there for a visit.

The horse Cyndie rode was named Buster. He was a gentle nag, but he had a tendency to stop to admire and eat the flowers. Whenever he would stop, the southern cowgirl in charge of the ride would yell, "Kick him in the boo-ute."

We must have heard that at least 20 times on the ride. To the point where "kick him in the boo-ute" has become an in-house joke among us.

Thinking of horses, I also remember Lady, resident of an acre pasture beside my home when Elaine and I first moved to Auburn. Lady and I had this cookie affair going. It started one day when I offered her a cookie and it went on for three years because she would not condone my passing the pasture without paying my cookie toll.

No matter where Lady was in that pasture, the minute I approached the fence she invariably ambled over to me and confidently waited for her handout. What I liked best was that she always seemed to perk up when I came onto the scene; I seemed to help make her day.

Our affair would probably still be going on except for the fact that pasture was converted to residential lots and Lady took up residence in another town. All this was a dozen or more years ago and Lady has since joined Prince in the heavenly pastures. But, just as with Prince, her memory lingers and it never fails to generate a smile.

Seems that about as close as I get to horses these days is reading a Dick Francis novel.

There was a little confusion near the end of our run because there was no sign indicating the Maryland border. We had a general idea because of the mileage, but we kept going, overrunning the distance, until we reached a sign reading, "Highway 332, Maryland."

In the short time we were in the state, I didn't learn much about Delaware. It was interesting, I thought, that the state got is name from Lord De La Warr, an early governor of Virginia.

I also learned that Wilmington, the largest city in the state, has a population of only 72,000. All the other 49 states have cities with a population larger than that. Yes, even Rhode Island, where Providence has a population of almost 161,000.

Seeing historic Port Penn was a pleasant voyage into history, and I did gain some understanding of how important the Delaware River was to the state's history and economy. Close my eyes and I can visualize the famous picture of George Washington crossing the Delaware one Christmas Eve to surprise the British and capture Trenton.

Other than for the nuisance of some heavy traffic at spots and of dealing at times with a shoulderless road, I had no problems with the romp across Delaware. I made a note to write to John Harvison and thank him for the route he suggested.

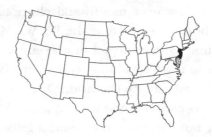

Chapter 12

New Jersey

Ticks, Strawberries and the Atlantic

Dates: *May 30th to June 2nd, 1997*
Miles: *57.4*
Route: *Start at Atlantic Ocean, Ocean City and follow city streets (36th Street, Central Avenue, 34th Street) to Highway 631. Take 631 west to Highway 50 and continue on 50 to junction with Highway 49. Follow 49 west to Salem, then take Tilbury Road, Sinnickson Landing Road to Sinnickson Landing and Delaware Bay, west boundary of New Jersey.*

DAY ONE. Leaving the sandy shores of the Atlantic Ocean and getting underway, I had a mile or so to navigate through built-up Ocean City. A helpful construction worker clued me that 34th Street was the key to exiting the town and getting onto our highway route.

Most of what I saw in Ocean City appeared to be tourist stuff. The place is overloaded with apartments, condos and motor courts – all wall to wall, all relatively new and all well maintained.

I felt lucky to get off the beach without being arrested because a sign told me that beach tags were required to be on the beach. In fact, the sign went on to specify that people were not permitted on the beach between 10 P.M. and six A.M., and prohibited on the beach or boardwalk at any time were dogs, picnicking, alcoholic beverages, open fires, loud music, ball or Frisbee throwing, and skateboards. Leaving the impression that this beach was a real fun place.

Amazingly I did not see a McDonald's on my way out of town, although a Dairy Queen was on the scene. A light mist was falling casting a moody shadow over me. To add cheer to my day and to refuel my ancient body, I stopped at the Wa Wa Market for a sourdough donut injection – almost an act of preventive medicine.

On the way out of town I had to negotiate one booby trap, a half-mile-long bridge over an estuary. The bridge had a two-lane road with a 20-inch shoulder. As cars zoomed toward me at 50 miles per hour, I knew I had better not trip, else I'd become a grille ornament.

In the middle of the bridge I came across a plaque dedicated to the memory of Cheryl M. Davis and Ronald J. Moretti, two teenagers killed by a drunk driver. My reaction: What this bridge needs is another plaque, one that reads, "Any drunk driver caught on this bridge will be forced to wear a 100-pound weight and then walk this bridge's plank leading to a 100-foot drop into the water."

On the north end of the bridge a young guy, probably around 25, handsome as Tom Cruise, was fishing. He had a cigarette dangling from his mouth.

I wanted to say, "Hey, life's too short already. Don't shorten it more. Get rid of that dirty, unhealthy habit."

But I kept my mouth shut. The strange part about it was that I felt somewhat guilty in doing so.

Once across the bridge I saw little but extensive marshlands for the next couple of miles. There were assorted businesses in the area where I crossed under the Garden Park Highway, an Interstate leading to New York City.

My day brightened when I came onto Highway 631 which had a breakdown lane – meaning no longer did I have to play tag with cars as I had done since leaving the Atlantic.

On prior visits to New Jersey I had seen only city and industrial areas. This area, with heavy forestation extending to both sides of the two-lane road, was a sharp contrast.

A sign told me I was in Cape May County, and the upper scale homes told me that this was an affluent area. Another conclusion I reached: In Montana if there's no dog in the back of your pickup, you're not a native. Here if there's no boat in your yard, you're not a native.

Got the idea, too, as I went past Resurrection Catholic Church advertising four masses on Sunday and two on Saturday, that the area has a substantial Catholic population. Wouldn't recommend putting a birth-control clinic here.

Another population that Elaine and I were beginning to notice as substantial was that of ticks. They were invading the dogs and us, flashing in our minds neon signs reading, "Lyme disease."

Every time I enter the motorhome for a pit stop, I am surprised to see so much crud on the front of my dark glasses, which I always wash at each stop. Nice to see this stuff on the glasses instead of feeling it in my eyes. I wear the glasses every bit as much to keep the crud out of my eyes as I do to keep the sun glare out.

The only city I passed through this first day after leaving Ocean City was Tuckahoe. On the south end of town the residences I saw looked old and tired, in need of some revitalization. Most sit only 20 feet or so off the road.

I passed by a diner, beauty shop, feed store and gas station without so much as a second look. But I braked suddenly when I saw the Tuckahoe Cheese Cake Factory.

Covert Bailey, do forgive me, but visions of indulging engulfed me. From that to strategy: Can I persuade Elaine to stop here after we finish today?

My big adventure happened in Tuckahoe after we finished our 12.6-mile day (shortened by an 11 A.M. start). I needed a haircut and found a barber shop in town.

The first thing I noticed on entering the shop was the ridiculously low price, $4, for a haircut – just half of the going rate in my hometown. My second observation was the warm greeting of the proprietor, Joe Spina:

"Hello, sir, nice to see you. I'll be with you very soon, sir. I'm just finishing this customer."

Once I got into the chair, Joe's staccato conversation continued until the time I left. He began with the usual business of asking where I was from and all such.

After I answered, he told me, "I was originally from Reading, Pennsylvania. But I married a girl from nearby Woodbine, and she could not stand Reading, so we moved here. I love this area, no tornadoes, no snow, mild winters and a low tax rate."

He explained that the tax rate was low because some big local corporation contributed heavily to the economy.

I don't quite recall what prompted Joe to tell me about his military career. But tell me about it, he did – from his entering the

Army Air Force in 1942 at age 18 until his discharge after the war.

Maybe that's where he learned all the "sir" business, I thought, because the word must have punctuated his conversation at least 50 times during our visit. The way I was getting closely shorn, I suspected he also learned barbering in the military.

"I was in Fresno, California," Joe said, "and me and this buddy of mine hitchhiked to Los Angeles. A forest ranger picked us up and asked where we were going, and we told him the Stage Door Canteen. He said that was exactly where he was going, and then he drove us right to the front door.

"The door was opened by Cecil DeMille, and Lucille Ball was standing there and she gave me a big hug and a kiss on the cheek. Her hair was fiery red, and she was dynamic. I was surprised at what a short guy DeMille was."

DAY TWO. My first leg of the day began like so many first legs – straightening out the kinks in my armor, flushing out my asthma. Similar to yesterday, the road was lined with heavy forestation.

Damn thing is encroaching on my vintage, I thought, as I crossed a small bridge built in 1929. My bet was that it was built before Black Tuesday of that year.

At the first pit stop Elaine was parked near a cemetery and church claiming to have been established in 1792. History I like, constant reminders of my mortality I do not like. Many of the graves went back more than 100 years.

In today's rain Elaine and I became aware of a New Jersey traffic law to the effect that cars with their wipers on must also have their lights on. The traffic signs read, "Wipers on? Burn lights."

Speaking of rain, ah the times how they do change. When I was in the motorhome for the six-mile pit stop, a torrential rain began to fall.

Back in the days when I ran across the USA (hard to believe that was six years ago), I would have said, "Damn the torpedoes, full steam ahead," and left the motorhome to run. But not so today when I handled the situation by telling Elaine, "I'll just sit here and wait this one out." Damn creampuff!

A few distractions as I wandered down the road:

- A pet-grooming shop with the name "Tiny Tailwaggers" left me on the verge of gagging.

- Six shots fired from an the adjacent woods got my full attention.
- I estimated the sign on the Mannatico Creek Bridge to be 100 years old. Crossing the bridge, I mused: How many people ever stop to give thought to what an impediment a waterway like this was to early pioneer travel.
- A roadside sign called my attention to Holly Orchards, but I saw no fruit-laden trees tempting me to sample the local product.

Oh, the things Elaine does to make me happy, I thought, as I left the 12-mile pit stop with a firm grip on two pieces of chocolate fudge she had just made. Nice munching on the road. True, not as fortifying as a Power Bar but considerably more yummy.

The road leading into Millville was lined with trees and attractive homes located 20 or more yards off the road. Sitting in front of one place was a 1929 Model-T coupe with a small pickup bed extending from it. It was for sale and the asking price was $6900, leaving me to wonder what Henry Ford's reaction would be if he looked down on this scene from his eternal perch.

I went past a five-year-old boy playing in his front yard. He saw my fanny pack and asked if I had a gun in it.

"No gun," I said, "but I do have a recorder." Pulling it out, I added, "Do you want to hear yourself talk?"

He beamed a yes. Said his name was Brian and gave his age. When I played back what he said, he glowed.

About then his father came out the front door, acted as if I were about to abscond with the kid as he rode to the rescue. Left me thinking, what a mixed-up world when you can't even be kind to a youngster without being suspect.

Besides, the guy must be blind. Couldn't he see the halo around my head!

On the excursion through town I noticed that the city had a nice small park with a lake and a jogging path around it. As I progressed through town on Main Street (what else could it possibly be called!), I saw that most of the downtown business was on High Street.

In the downtown area, I crossed over Maurice River Bridge that was crowded with people fishing. Even though Millville is known as the "Holly City" from the many holly trees cultivated in the area, I failed to see any.

The nearest RV park after we finished our 17.2-mile day just north of Millville was 22 miles away. As we drove there on County Road 635, all we saw was acres and acres of agriculture. Good evidence of why New Jersey is called the "Garden State."

DAY THREE. My third day in New Jersey started on a somewhat blasphemous note. This being a Sunday, my thoughts at one point turned to church and religion.

My blasphemy resulted from seeing the Pope on CNN and hearing him tell people they should give to feed the poor. My immediate thought was, Just how much did the Papal treasury kick in?

Then another thought, this one heretical: Could it be that, purely out of their being inherently vain, people believe – without their even knowing or realizing it – that they are immortal? As vain as they are, they cannot conceive of their existing only for a lifetime and then dissolving into dust?

A depressing thought. I decided I must have read it somewhere, and only now did it resurrect from the buried recess of my mind.

I prefer the more buoyant thought that we are all creatures of God here on earth – on trial with God as judge and jury, and the verdict heaven or hell depending on how we lived our lives. This statement is heresy to Elaine and her Lutheran faith.

She claims that we are all creatures of God, doing our best to please Him, knowing we will fail in many ways. According to Elaine, if we believe in God, He will forgive us in spite of our inadequacies and welcome us to heaven when we die.

Enter the small-world department: On one of Elaine's pit stops she was parked in front of a home where the name on the mailbox read, "Roy Dan Reese." Like Billy Bob, Freddie Joe and all such, it sounded Texan to me.

While buying groceries at an IGA Market, Elaine witnessed a commentary on parenting or sociology, or both, hereabouts. As she was entering the market, a mother with her two sons was by the front door.

The mother asked them, "Do you have to pee?" They said, "Yes," and she told them to go ahead. So they stood beside the front door and cut loose, and in doing so commented on the velocity of their streams.

Elaine had to tippy toe in to avoid their puddles. Ye gods, no wonder teachers have trouble with discipline in the schools!

Upbeat day in that the sun appeared for the first time in three days. All kinds of good things happening in New Jersey, I was thinking. This just might be the first state I've crossed without seeing a snake.

But it's appropriate that the state should smack of good things. After all, it produced Edison who gave us the electric light bulb; Morse who invented the telegraph, and Holland who invented the parachute.

Edison and Morse I already knew about, but how could I wear a parachute so many months in combat and not know that Holland invented it? Sorry for being so ungrateful, John. Associatively I wondered if this is the same Holland after whom the Holland Tunnel was named.

Besides producing inventors, New Jersey hosted the first organized baseball game (Hoboken, 1846) and the first intercollegiate football game (New Brunswick, 1869) A couple events not covered by ABC Sports.

It took about three miles for me to work my way through Bridgeton, the second-largest city (population about 19,000) on our New Jersey route. Again, even though I was still on Highway 49, the main drag was unimaginatively named Main Street and the newest building in town was a state office building at Main and Canal Streets.

After crossing the Cohansey River in the middle of town, I saw a formidable-looking building which turned out to be the Cumberland County Jail. The adjacent Cumberland Courthouse resembled Independence Hall in Philadelphia (or, if you prefer, its replica at Knott's Berry Farm in California).

The building that impressed me the most was the Ebenezer Miller/Andrew Hunter home dating back to 1759. Hope I don't offend many people by saying that every time I see the name Ebenezer, I have trouble believing it is for real.

The historic Broad Street Presbyterian Church – founded in 1792, a two-story brick building surrounded by a cemetery – was no kid itself.

I can't ever recall seeing a larger middle school than the one I saw in Bridgeton. For a moment I thought this three-story brick building, about 150 yards on each of its rectangular sides, might be the local Pentagon.

For good reason much of what I saw in Bridgeton appeared to be old. The city has more than 2200 homes and buildings on the National Historic Register.

Two things in New Jersey remained constant for us today. Ticks were as plentiful as smokers in a gambling casino, and strawberries were for sale every couple of miles.

There was nothing distinctive about the two small communities, Hopewell and Shiloh, I went through after leaving Bridgeton. Hopewell was home to fast-food places, a gas station, pizza joint, a deli and the Cumberland Insurance Group headquarters. Sort of a sad commentary that Shiloh, where the homes sit only 15 feet or so off the road and which dates all the way back to 1705, has failed to come up with anything distinctive.

The biggest operation hereabouts is the De Cou Orchards. Located four miles west of Bridgeton on Route 49, the farm grows peaches, nectarines, apples, grapes, pumpkins and berries.

The farm offers seniors a special deal: Buy one basket of fruit, and get another free. I had to pass because I was in no mood to lug two baskets of fruit down the road. I had my hands full just moving one ancient body down the road, albeit I was having no running problems as I moved along at a leisurely pace while absorbing the passing scene.

We finished a 16.7-mile day about eight miles south of Salem and then made our usual long drive to an RV park.

DAY FOUR. Nasty as our fourth and final New Jersey day started– rain and a 20-mile-per-hour crosswind. I was more than glad that I had only a little more than eight miles to run.

Near Quinton I read the only historical marker I saw in New Jersey. It related to the Revolutionary War and marked a spot where the Colonials, at a loss of seven men, held the line against the British. Seemed to me that, at the very least, the marker could have named the seven men who gave their lives here.

Coming into Salem, I thought, Just how many Salems are there in the USA? Let's see, I could think of Salem, Massachusetts, and witch-craft; Salem, Missouri, and friend Ray Vickery who owns a newspaper there; Salem, Oregon, where a distant relative lives; Salem, Arkansas, near the home of my friend Ray Mahannah; Salem, Kentucky, seen on our driving this summer; Salem, South Dakota, driven through when we were running the state last summer; and probably a half-dozen others unknown to me.

My second thought in Salem was, Be careful on these sidewalks. The walks, made of brick and somewhat wavy, presented the danger of tripping or stumbling.

This was on my mind because twice I've fallen on bumpy sidewalks and cracked my forehead, and the result was some MD practicing his stitching on me. Never will forget the name of the first: Dr. Turnipseed, and a good stitcher he was.

I paused at the south end of Salem to study a two-story brick home named the Matthew Keasbey home, built in 1817. Nothing else attractive did I see in my 2.5-mile jaunt through Salem, despite the city's population of 65,000. The city's attractions lay elsewhere than my route.

The town did appear to have an inordinate number of black people, by my estimate 70 percent of the people I saw were black.

The sight of a fossil jogging through town drew a number of broad smiles as well as a number of waves and "Hi's." One youngster wanted to know, "Where did you come from?"

I was tempted to tell him I was an alien. Instead I kept it in terms he would understand: "Oh, I'm just jogging through this town."

I was afraid that if I said, "I started from the Atlantic Ocean." The next move would have been to give him a lesson in geography.

Out of Salem we headed for Sinnickson's Landing on the Delaware Bay, marking the western coast of New Jersey and termination of our east-west run from the Atlantic Ocean. All told our route covered 57.4 miles.

The run over, I asked Elaine, "Well, what do you remember most about New Jersey?"

"The ticks," she replied. "Seems I was picking them off Rebel, Brudder and us all of the time."

"How about you?" she asked. "What do you remember most?"

"Well, the thing I saw the most was strawberries for sale about every two miles," I told her. "Two dollars a basket."

So saying, I was reminded of the unattended roadside stand where the owner had baskets of strawberries and a coffee can for depositing money. That guy goes much beyond, "In God we trust."

With Elaine reflecting on ticks and my reflecting on strawberries, New Jersey could hardly be called a cultural experience. Maybe we will get some of that in New England, I thought, as we headed in that direction. Going north, I hoped that the running in New England would be as easy as the romp across New Jersey.

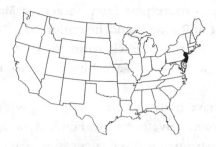

Chapter 13

Rhode Island

Lost in Providence

Dates: *June 4th and 5th, 1997*
Miles: *32.4*
Route: *Start on Highway 14 in Connecticut and follow it into Rhode Island and its junction with 14/102. Continue on 14/102 into Providence. Cross Point Street Bridge, follow city streets to Red Bridge, and cross Seekonk River and get onto Highway 44, which leads to Massachusetts/Rhode Island border.*

DAY ONE. There's some irony here, I thought as I lined up to start running across Rhode Island. This is the smallest state in the nation – in fact, it's sometimes called "Little Rhody" – and yet I will run farther across it than I've run across some larger states. A second irony is that it is known as the "Ocean State," yet nowhere on my route will I see the ocean.

My original plan to cross Rhode Island called for me to run either Highway 44 or Highway 138, west to east. This plan got scratched when Edmond T. Parker, Chief Civil Engineer for the Rhode Island Department of Transportation, told me, "These are probably the last routes we would suggest, they are high-speed roadways with very high auto and truck volumes and inconsistent shoulder widths."

Mr. Parker suggested that I follow Highway 14 west to east across the state, then cross the Seekonk River and proceed to the Massachusetts border. I owe the guy a heap of thanks for steering me to a pleasant route, albeit my excursion through Providence was a traffic nightmare.

When I ran this route past Dave Sargent, a Marine Corps class-mate and resident of Rhode Island, he endorsed it. Back in our officer candidate days Dave tried to elicit sympathy from me because of the problems the name "Sargent" gave him as he went through officer training.

But I would have none of that, countering with, "How'd you like to be the very next guy to follow Frank X. Reagan, All-American halfback at Pennsylvania for three successive years, in every physical action we do–like throwing a hand grenade, charging down a bayonet course, scaling an obstacle course."

Reagan's shadow fell on me up to the very moment that I was commissioned. As we went singly across the stage to receive our commissions, the national newsreels were filming Reagan. Just as I started to move on stage, an officer restrained me so that there would be no distraction from the Reagan filming. I was told to move on stage only after Reagan had cleared it.

After the long drive from New Jersey, during which Elaine skirted the Philadelphia and New York City environs to avoid heavy traffic, I was somewhat indisposed to running. On the drive we enjoyed a beautiful journey up the Delaware River in Buck's County, seeing some lovely estates, and we got to see the Catskills, the closest we'd ever been before was to see this area as a setting for movies such as "Dirty Dancing."

Today started with an unusual experience that happened as we were leaving the RV park. As I was putting a garbage bag in a dumpster, I found myself eyeball to eyeball with a raccoon that was down among the garbage.

Seeing me, he backed into a corner and cowered. Seeing him, I backed away from the dumpster.

Later as Elaine and I talked about the encounter, we wondered if the animal had jumped into the dumpster for food and then found himself with no way of climbing out. I regretted not thinking of that when I saw the raccoon because I would have put a board into the dumpster so that he could walk out on it.

Seeing him set me to thinking back on some of the raccoons I had seen on my uncle's ranch. They were three-legged raccoons because they had been trapped and in order to escape they had bitten off their trapped leg.

Arriving at our Rhode Island start on Highway 14, we could not locate a state boundary marker, and for good reason since there was none. The map told us that the junction of Highway 14 and Highway 14A was in Connecticut, a bit to the west of the Rhode Island/Connecticut border, so just to make sure we didn't miss any of Rhode Island we started at that junction on a cloudy, rain-threatening afternoon.

Once underway I confirmed my suspicion about being indisposed to running. Even jogging was a strain after a couple of days of motorhome, traveling and rump-residing.

Very soon, though, my mind began to focus on the tranquility and rural beauty of the setting. The large homes, some of respectable vintage, were attractive and of contrasting designs.

Many homes, I noticed, were painted a rust color that made the surrounding colorful foliage all the more resplendent. One stone home, built in 1826, was very remindful of Anne Hathaway's cottage in England, albeit no reminders of William Shakespeare were about.

If Robert Frost were correct with his line "Good fences make good neighbors," there must be a lot of good neighbors in these parts because I was seeing stone fences all along the route. Ever the prosaic one, I wondered how many man hours were spent in collecting these stones and then in stacking them into fences. They were the only type of fences seen, and I guessed that might be dictated by some sort of ordinance.

The homes in the first eight miles or so were spaced about 80 to 100 yards apart, and in every direction I looked I saw an abundance of pine trees. The oldest home I saw was the Thomas Brown house, dating back to 1770.

Newly painted a rosy rust color and excellently maintained, this two-story frame house's age was evident only from the plaque adorning it. Who was this guy Thomas Brown to have such an elegant pad as this back in the 1700s, I wondered?

I got the distinct impression that people in this area were concerned about crime, even thought Rhode Island ranks 33rd among states in crimes reported. A "Private Property, Keep Out" sign was posted on most homes. Some had signs reading, "Doberman Guard Dog on Duty."

One sign pictured two Dobermans and the words, "We can make

it to the fence in three seconds. Can you?"

The question I had in passing was not how fast the dogs could make it to the fence. It was, Are they ever inclined to jump over it?

The only dog incident I had today was when a Boxer charged out from one home toward me. I picked up a stick and he retreated, lovable coward that he was.

When I came to the junction of Highway 14 and Highway 102 south, the setting changed. This area had less forestation, more open space, but the homes continued to be upscale.

The name on a gated driveway I went past reminded me of an officer I knew in the Marine Corps. A major, he was assigned to work for a friend of mine, John Stevens, a lieutenant colonel commanding an infantry battalion.

John was an outstanding officer and he expected – better yet, *demanded* – excellence of his officers. The major, fearful of working for John, faked an illness and worked his way into a desk job at regimental headquarters, even though the job was actually a captain's billet.

The major did a masterful job of brown-nosing the regimental commander. And the irony here is that, between his habitual brown-nosing and avoiding responsibility, he went on to make colonel, whereas John – an officer of more knowledge and integrity – resigned, largely for personal reasons, as a lieutenant colonel.

I had it on direct testimony from a friend in higher headquarters that this major was involved in the deliberate loss (i.e., destroying) of a fitness report highly complimentary to an officer. The regimental commanding officer did not want to see him receiving a complimentary report.

Most drivers today were considerate by moving over as they approached me. Yet nary a one returned my wave of thanks. Seemed contradictory.

Went past a church with a sign, "Repent and believe in the gospel." This raised in my mind the question, What about repenting and not believing in the gospel?

A conversation with Helen Knight offered a change from my solitary meditation. We met when she was picking up mail from her mailbox.

When I first saw her and as we talked she reminded me of Sister Marion Irvine, a superb athlete who at age 54 qualified for the

Olympic Marathon Trial. Both ladies are in their 60s, gray-haired, tall and athletic, quick on the mental trigger and full of life.

In the course of our conversation when I asked about winter weather, Helen told me, "We sometimes have 20 inches of snow here in the winter. That's not common, but it does happen."

"What does it get in degrees?" I asked.

"Oh gosh, it gets cold," she replied. "Ten to 14 degrees below zero. And as you can see, we also have a lot of heat and humidity in the summer."

Helen pretty much characterized the area I was in when she said, "When you live in this rural area, you really don't want to go into town very much."

At the junction of Highways 14 east, 94 north, and 102 north I studied a monument dedicated to Gaento del Giudice that told me he lived from 1887 to 1972, that he was known as the "Man with the horn," that he was a veteran of World War I and a founder of the American Legion. Only thing I remembered about the founding of the Legion was that Alexander Woollcott was one of the founders, or at least I think he was.

Prior to starting today's outing in Rhode Island, I had no particular expectations of what I would see. Yet I was caught off guard seeing the proliferation of pine trees and stone fences – the latter, by my guess, having been in place in many instances since colonial times. Encountering a few hills along the way also came as a surprise.

Another unexpected happening came about when I found myself running down a hill at a fairly good clip. I felt blessed to be able to do so because at three A.M. I struggled through an asthma attack that had me gasping for each breath.

The miracle or mystery of it is that once the attack is over, a process than can last an agonizing hour or more, and I begin to get a certain amount of breathing equilibrium, I am subsequently able to recover to the point of being able to run. Blissful when that happens!

I really didn't feel like quitting at 11 miles, but considering our late-afternoon start we had done well to get that far. Besides, we faced the task of locating an RV facility in this area where such were sparse.

DAY TWO. Driving to the start today, I reflected on one tidbit I learned last night about Rhode Island. Though the smallest state it has the longest official name: the "State of Rhode Island and Providence Plantations."

I also reflected on the fact that the RV park where we stayed last night would accept only cash payments – no credit cards or checks. Smacked of a bit of IRS hanky-panky to me.

Again I started in a pleasant rural setting, with big estates in evidence. Looking through the gates of one, I saw that the grounds were as large as three football fields.

Three times during the first five miles I had to negotiate my way on a causeway over a reservoir. The problem here was that the road had but two lanes with a guard rail on each side and no shoulder of any kind.

My only option here when a car approached was to sit on the rail and bend my legs and feet under it. The wind was strong enough to white-cap the reservoir water and to blow my ball cap off a couple of times.

By the time I reached the junction of Highway 116, this a little past five miles, I had trudged up a couple of hills, one a mile long. At the junction Suzy Q's Ice Cream and Hamburger Stand appeared to be doing a brisk business.

Bill's garage had nearly 100 cars parked around it, but I saw no action. Could Bill be that far behind in his workload?

A nearby sign read, "Welcome to the town of Johnson, Inc. March 6, 1759." From what little I saw, I concluded Johnson must have gone into hibernation since incorporating.

Around six miles I became aware that the sun was jitterbugging around dark clouds, causing me to fret about getting drenched. At the same time I noticed – who could miss that stench? – that every fourth vehicle passing me was a garbage truck on its way to the nearby city dump.

I got a good fix on my location when I passed under I-295. Emerging from the underpass, I did a double-take at a pasture and saw grazing there half a dozen of the largest sheep I've ever seen. This pastoral scene was unexpected.

Little did I realize when I met with Elaine for a pit stop at eight miles that this would be the last time I'd see her for more than three hours. This was the result of our getting separated in Providence and not joining up again until we reached Massachusetts.

Shortly after leaving the pit stop, I was jolted from the serenity of serene, almost resorty, Rhode Island to the hurly-burly of greater Providence environs. From the time I crossed Highway 5 until I reached Massachusetts, I was immersed in trying to avoid getting hit by a car, trying at times to avoid some unsavory characters and trying (somewhat unsuccessfully) to keep reasonably oriented on where I was and where I was going.

Going by a rundown shopping district, a little more than nine miles into my day, I began to realize I was not in the best of neighborhoods. By 12 miles I realized that Elaine and I were separated with neither of us having the least idea of where the other was.

By now I had to run the sidewalks since there was no space for me on the two lanes of fast moving traffic. In the residential areas house fronts were directly on the sidewalk, many people were about, and I found the passage slow and laborious as I dodged people. It got so bad that at one point I had to stop at a McDonald's and fortify myself with a freshly baked apple turnover.

In one ricky-ticky business area I passed through I had the experience of witnessing two different drug deals going down. No way was I tempted to make a citizen's arrest!

One dealer was kneeling on the sidewalk talking with the occupants of a car. I passed within three feet of them, but they paid no attention to me.

I never saw so many $20 bills in one hand as that dealer held. I could hear him dickering over price.

I had anticipated that when I reached the central Providence area I would be able to follow the sketch map I carried and work my way across the Seekonk River, and from there to the Massachusetts border. Instead I ran into what one writer called "a confusing ganglia of roads, canals, and freeways all intertwined."

As if that were not enough, some of the streets were blocked off. If I recall correctly, this was because Hillary Clinton was in the area.

And in another area, traffic was being rerouted because the fire department was putting out a small fire. There was a plethora of one-way streets and many of the streets ran at tangents and some were without street signs.

Entering this mass of confusion, I did get a good look at the Regency Plaza, the Holiday Inn, and the Providence skyline – most notably the towering Industrial National Bank Building and the Hospital Trust Tower. I kept thinking that Providence seemed bigger than its reported population of approximately 161,000.

Couldn't help but wonder which areas of this city Roger Williams frequented and exactly where he first came ashore. Williams came to Providence in 1636 when he was exiled from Puritan Massachusetts for his religious views that included the separation of church and state, and his belief that the Indians should be paid for their lands. Despite his beliefs it seemed that he conveniently forgot to pay the Narragansett Indians for land in Rhode Island.

In my wandering in the central area of Providence, absorbed as I was with trying to find my way, I failed to see any colonial-era houses though Providence has more than any other city. I did not get a glimpse of prestigious Brown University, and not even a good look at the state capitol. Nor did I see Providence's indoor shopping center that is, so I learned, the oldest one in the nation.

Wandering about, sometimes even retracing my steps and adding extra mileage, I was beginning to feel like an NFL quarterback who had forgotten his play book. Not only was I failing navigation, but missing so many tourist attractions, I was failing tourism.

One detour took me down a colorful street – I think the name was Wickenham or Wickendam – of small cafes, coffee houses, trendy dress shops, flower shops, music stores and such. A barber shop advertised haircuts for $15, almost double the going rate in my hometown. At that rate, I concluded coffee must be $3 a cup.

The only building I entered was a public library, where my shorts and T-shirt attire raised a few eyebrows. I was not there by choice but rather to answer the call of my demanding bladder.

As I kept trudging along, not even stopping for food or drink but simply rationing my eight ounces of water and munching on a Power Bar, I kept worrying about Elaine and how we would rendezvous. My hope was that once I crossed the bridge over the Seekonk River, I'd find her on the other side. If not there, at the Massachusetts border where we had agreed to meet if we got separated.

I was stopped at a street corner, studying my sketch map to confirm that I was headed for the bridge, when Donna Barry passing by, noticed my look of concern and asked if she could help. And that she did by confirming that I was indeed headed in the right direction and that the bridge was a little over a half-mile away.

I thanked her profusely and in the course of our subsequent conversation she told me, "I stopped because I saw your T-shirt – 'Running Across All 50 States' – and I wanted to know if that was true." Whereupon I briefed her on our expedition.

In turn she told me, "I'm a mother and a real estate agent" I liked that billing; she had her priorities right.

After extra miles, much confusion and lost time in Providence, I came upon what Donna called the Red Bridge that crossed the Seekonk River. Once I crossed the bridge and arrived in East Providence, I took a quick look around for Elaine.

Not finding her, I successfully navigated my way to Highway 44 that led to the Massachusetts border. The streets leading to 44, and 44 itself, were jammed with fast-moving traffic.

When I arrived at the Massachusetts border, clearly marked with a sign, Elaine was not to be seen. I made several attempts to locate or stop a trucker with a CB who could contact her.

That failing, I thought, How in hell do I tell her where I am? The question no sooner asked than Alexander Graham Bell rode to my rescue.

"Phone her," he said. I added another mile to my day before I was able to locate a phone. I dialed our cell-phone number, and the call was processed back to Auburn, California (our cell-phone home base), then relayed back to Elaine at her cell phone in Rhode Island.

Once we connected, we discovered we were only two miles apart – she at the Massachusetts border on Highway 152, I at the border on Highway 44. While she was driving to join up with me, I adjourned to the adjacent McDonald's and over coffee reflected on how our planning had gone awry.

Anticipating that we might get separated in the Providence environs, we had agree that our rendezvous point would be at the Rhode Island/Massachusetts border. The problem was that we did not study the map closely enough to realize that on the east side of the Seekonk bridge *two* roads lead to the border, Highways 152 and 44. Unfortunately one of us followed 152 and the other 44.

The lesson here for the future: Double-check my map reading. Probably would be a good idea, too, if we avoided traffic jigsaw puzzles like Providence. Nice town, but I wouldn't want to drive there!

Elaine agrees that she doesn't ever want to drive in Providence again. After being stuck in the bricked street downtown area, in a motorhome, during a rally of some sort and being totally lost among the one-way streets, her nerves were shot. "If it hadn't been for the courteous and helpful drivers, I wouldn't have made it," she said. "Rhode Island should get the award for patient and courteous drivers."

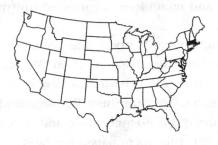

Chapter 14

Massachusetts

A Pilgrim's Progress

Dates: *June 6th to 8th, 1997*
Miles: *39.8*
Route: *Start at east border of Massachusetts, Cape Cod Bay, Plymouth, and follow Highway 44 west all the way to Providence and Rhode Island border.*

DAY ONE. Our original battle plan for Massachusetts was to run Highway 7, north from the Vermont border south to the Connecticut border. A plan embellished when Kevin J. Sullivan, commissioner of the Massachusetts Highway Department, told me, this "is probably the shortest and most scenic route you will find to traverse across our beautiful state."

Julius E. Goldblatt, a resident of Lexington, Massachusetts and a Marine Corps classmate, also endorsed the route. I admire Julius because after World War II he went back to school to become an MD, just as classmate George Teller did. How can I help but admire guys like that who, after three years of warfare, submit themselves to the rigors of medical school?

Another assurance I had that Highway 7 was a feasible route came from Katherine Kiefer, a runner and an attorney now residing in Lexington. Having run ultra races with her in California, I knew her judgment was sound.

So informed, I was primed to run Highway 7 across the state. But as Robert Burns told us a couple hundred years ago, the best laid schemes of mice and men often get messed up (more precisely, he said, "Gang aft a-gley").

And that's exactly what happened as we ran Rhode Island and I suddenly noticed that the distance from Massachusetts' western border at Rhode Island to Massachusetts' eastern border at Plymouth Bay was only 40 miles. After finishing Rhode Island, we'd be on the scene and could drive this 40-mile route and check it for feasibility. The net result after this reconnaissance was a decision to run Highway 44 east from Plymouth Bay to the Rhode Island border.

How could I tread more on history, find a more suitable site to begin a run across Massachusetts than where the Pilgrims first set foot ashore in 1620? By actual account 102 came ashore here, the same number that started the 66-day voyage from England – but not exactly the same people because en route one had died and one was born.

The newborn – maybe appropriately but not too desirably, I'd suspect – was given the first name of Oceanus. Maybe Oceanus didn't have to live with that name very long, though, because half the pilgrims died during the severe winter and it is likely, being an infant, that Oceanus was among them.

Arriving in Plymouth and getting underway, Elaine and I did not linger very long in the area because we'd been there a couple years prior on a Tauck Tour and had seen the sights. I did pause long enough to photograph Plymouth Rock and the Mayflower II.

The rock, which has 1620 carved into it and is about the size of a well-fed Iowa hog, supposedly marks the spot where the Pilgrims first set foot. The rock is protected by a granite portico resembling a Greek temple.

The Mayflower II is a full-scale reproduction of the original Mayflower, a three-masted merchant vessel. The II actually sailed from England to Plymouth in 44 days in 1957 (that, I hastily add, to spare any calculators going into action, is 22 days faster than the voyage of the original Mayflower).

From our previous visit we knew that one of the best attractions in the area is about three miles out of town. This is Plymouth Plantation, which faithfully resembles the complete village of 1627.

The village is staffed with people costumed as Pilgrims and behaving as they did then. For example, their vocabulary and knowledge extend only to what was known at the time they "lived."

These Pilgrims are busy cooking, gardening, making and repairing equipment, tending to animals – but they will interrupt their chores to answer questions from visitors. The place is authentic to the point of having animals and chickens (visitor, be careful where you step!). Adjacent to the Plantation is the Wampanoag Indian Settlement which gives an insight into how the Indians lived.

Leaving the Bay, bidding fond adieu to Plymouth Rock and following Water Street, I took notice that the Bay was dotted with small craft, that Water Street was lined with motels/hotels, souvenir shops and an array of parking meters. Too much tacky stuff in such a historic setting, I thought.

Once out of the waterfront I was on a narrow, two-lane street with houses and businesses interspersed on both sides of the road. Surprising how many old homes had been converted as offices for CPA's, MD's, DDS's, attorneys, insurance agents and even a car-rental business.

Even though I had to negotiate a hill of a mile or so and of six-percent gradient, most of it on a sidewalk my egress from the Bay was fairly comfortable. Once atop the hill I looked around full circle and saw heavy forestation everywhere I looked.

Miles Standish is big in these parts, I concluded, after passing the Miles Standish Memorial, Miles Standish Shopping Plaza and Miles Standish State Park. Miles, why am I having trouble recalling your role here? About all I can resurrect is that – if I can believe Longfellow's poem – is that, choked up over proposing to Priscilla Mullens, you had to persuade John Alden to ask her on your behalf.

Funny thing, Miles, in the three years I went to high school with a kid named Miles Cosgrove, I never once gave thought to whether he might be named after you, and now here I am musing over that possibility. My most vivid memory of Miles Cosgrove is that, just like the mile record-holder Glenn Cunningham, his legs were burned while he was a child.

Yet, again like Cunningham, he excelled at long-distance running. I should know because I got a good rear view of him as he lead me down many a road.

About three miles from the Bay area the sidewalk disappeared and I ran into tough sledding – a 12-inch paved shoulder, bumper-to-bumper-traffic. It was not all bad, though, because when I stepped off the road to avoid approaching cars, I stepped on the sand, which was better than tall grass where I can't see where I am stepping.

At this point most of the homes along the route are upper middle class. If I saw the price tag, I might be labeling them luxurious.

Here, as in Rhode Island, Delaware and New Jersey, I saw in the front and back yards of many homes statues of the Blessed Virgin Mary. Come to think of it, in all my travels in California, I can't recall seeing even one statue to the BVM.

Around five miles I thought, Now there's a first, as I read a sign, "Caution: Deaf Person."

At the six-mile pit stop Elaine was parked by some cranberry fields. I was able to recognize them as such only because of having been shown some during a Tauck Tour of this area.

Nonetheless this knowledge did give me, a fugitive from botany, somewhat of a superior feeling. The berries grow in low-lying bogs, and when the bogs are flooded (in September and October), Ocean Spray stockholders are treated to the sight of lakes of brilliant red cranberries.

Around seven miles I came upon a newly surfaced road with a bike lane. The jubilation of this is akin to Lewis and Clark being appreciative of a swift current carrying their canoes downstream.

By now I was aware of some splendid examples of Cape Code architecture along this road. I was also taking notice of the heavy forestation on both sides of the road and the fact that only 20 percent of the drivers moved over to give me running space.

In North Carver I ducked into a cavernous building called the Book Barn to see if I could find a running book not in my collection of 450 such books. I was lucky enough to latch onto one.

At eight miles the junction of Highways 44 and 58 was typical of so many road junctions in having a number of gas stations, convenience stores, and of course the Golden Arches. Going past Honey Dew Donuts, I felt inclined to indulge but, alas, I had squandered all my cash at the Book Barn.

Francis Bacon told us, "Some books are to be tasted, others to be swallowed, and some few to be chewed and digested." All I can say is that having cost me a gooey donut or two, the book I bought better be in the "digested" category.

Around nine miles an amusement area, highly patronized, grabbed my attention. It was a smorgasbord of batting cages, go carts, miniature golf, bumper car rides, a video arcade and nearby a golf driving range to keep dad busy while the kids went berserk. As I passed, I could hear the cash registers clicking.

It was refreshing, at 9.5 miles, to be out of the built-up area and on a two-lane highway with a breakdown lane on each side. Elated, I felt like doing a Richard Simmons goody-goody dance but resisted since I am on an energy conservation program.

A sign I seldom see on my state crossings told me I was approaching a rotary with six spokes. While running the London-to-Brighton race and encountering such a roundabout, we never knew beforehand which was the exit spoke. So we had to run, watch cars and scout for a chalk mark on the outside of the spoke – which required 20/20 vision because the British were frugal with chalk to the point of where one barely perceptible mark was almost an extravagance.

Just prior to coming into the motorhome for the 12-mile pit stop, I saw an oversized truck with a pilot car approaching and taking half the breakdown lane, so I scooted to the adjacent bushes and watched them pass. When I came into the motorhome, Elaine said, "I hear you almost got hit by a truck."

"What do you mean? I ran out into the boondocks because they were crowding the breakdown lane, and I watched them pass."

"Well," she said, "here's what they said on the CB. 'That old guy looks like he's taking a risk. He looks like he's almost 90 and like he needs a rest. Or maybe a rest home.'" Then Elaine added, "Love it, love it."

Hell, I was standing still. If I'd been in motion, they might have said 100.

To quote Rodney Dangerfield (cheez, how desperate can I get!), "I get no respect." Even at 80 I'd be willing to wager that truck driver $50 that I could beat him in a mile race.

If he wants to go three miles, I'll raise the wager to $100. A thousand if he so much as mentions a marathon! We'll see who looks 90, said the sensitive one!

To the state's credit I should mention that two drivers braked and were backing up to offer me help when I waved them on.

An unexpected development when I came to a divided highway and saw a sign, "Bicycles, scooters and pedestrians prohibited." Doesn't make sense, I thought; this is a divided highway, much safer than what I've been running.

Without so much as a second thought, into the valley of a possible traffic citation I charged. Actually there was no other option if I wanted to get to the Rhode Island border.

Kind of encouraging a few minutes later to have a bicyclist pass me, doing about 25 miles per hour. With a 10-foot breakdown lane and a 50-MPH speed limit, prohibiting pedestrians here is ridiculous. But after seeing that sign, I ran the last four miles like a man possessed while trying to get off this road without being arrested.

One thing I could not complain about today was the weather: temperature in the low 70s, no wind, very comfortable for running. A day we did not take full advantage of because, humoring my antiquity, we folded at 16.4 miles.

DAY TWO. If my bookkeeping is correct, I thought this morning, we've been on the road 329 days all told jogging across states. I have yet to miss a day because of sickness.

Today was about as close as I've come because last night I had an upset stomach, diarrhea and no energy. I felt lucky to resurrect and to be back on the road this morning.

As I moved along my first mile, I had the uneasy feeling that I might have a confrontation with a state trooper ordering me off the road. Luckily that did not materialize, most likely because I had less than two miles to do on this road. Once I reached the I-495 area and negotiated the rotary there, relying on all my London-to-Brighton skills to do so, I left the restricted road and got onto a two-lane highway bedecked with forestation, businesses or residences.

Now instead of worrying about getting arrested I could fret about some careless driver descending on me. The irony here was that I was now legally running on a road that has a small bike lane, less than half the protection that the breakdown lane on the restricted road afforded me. In other words, in the place where I had the most protection, it was illegal to run.

Around 2.5 miles I came into Lakeville, incorporated in 1853 – a mere child around here compared to some of the other stuff around here. Taunton, for instance, was established in 1639.

Waiting to cross a street, I heard a man standing beside me say, "What charity are you running for?"

"None really," I replied. "I don't have any sponsor."

His question did not surprise me because one of the first questions I usually get is, "Who's sponsoring you?" or, "Who's paying you for this run?" or, "What charity are you running for?" All being a reflection of American materialism, the Yankee dollar on the march again. The majority of people have difficulty believing Elaine and I are out here for the sheer enjoyment of it.

I paused a moment to study the Taunton River – about 15 feet wide, lined with trees to the water's edge and indeed an accurate barometer of my age. As a kid I would have had the urge to plunge into it; as a fossil, I'm simply content to jog across the bridge.

Once I did so, a sign told me I was in Raynham, incorporated in 1731. By now I was aware that I was seeing all kinds of town signs but not seeing the business sections of the towns themselves, all of which seem to be located to the north or south of Highway 44.

One distinctive feature of Raynham was a series of car dealerships located along the highway. Also prominent in Raynham was that octopus of merchandising known as Wal Mart. Enough to make a Pilgrim roll over in his grave.

Down the road a short distance was a shopping center with 20 or more stores and traffic so thick it took me five minutes to get across the street. While waiting I read a sign telling me that downtown Raynham was one mile to the north.

As I came into the outskirts of downtown Taunton, I was completely confused as to how the different town boundaries were delineated. I'd seen a Taunton sign, then a Raynham sign and now here I was in the town of Taunton itself.

With almost 50,000 residents it was no hamlet. It took me almost two miles to work my way through the town while being treated to several diversions along the way. The first was a gingerbread house with a big sign reading, "Evolution is life. Creation is the fruit. (Genesis Ch 1, Verse 1)." Parked in the home's yard were a red Wrangler and a Saab convertible, both of which sent mixed signals to me because they didn't seem to jibe with a biblical quote.

Over one stretch of three blocks I did some serious gawking at several three-story homes, each of interesting architecture, that were the size of small hotels. Going through the downtown, I saw traffic blocked off in front of the city hall and had to study the situation to determine the occasion was a Cinco de Mayo celebration.

About the time I reached the town square, a pleasant small park with a statue of an infantry World War I soldier in it, the traffic was horrendous – worst met in 13 states run to date this year, except for the Providence maze.

Thinking of Providence and being lost reminded me of a race I'd run 10 years or more ago in Nevada City, California, in company with Walt Lange and Pete Hansen, among others. Realizing that the newly fallen snow might cover course markings, I memorized the route. I was running at the tail end of the lead group at a point where the course swung left but the lead group had mistakenly turned right.

Confidently turning left, I yelled to Walt and Pete ahead of me. They retreated, and the three leaders in the race now were Walt, Pete and me. Good Lord, I thought, with a little less than two miles to go we could win this race if the lead group does not get turned around on time.

About then while rounding a corner, I again saw Pete headed in the wrong direction and I yelled to him. Catching me and passing, he was muttering, "Son of a bitch, son of a bitch."

Meanwhile Walt was moving fast and sensing a possible victory. But not Pete; he took another wrong turn and once again I had to call him back.

I knew he was passing me again when I heard behind me, "Son of a bitch, son of a bitch."

Just when I was catching sight of the finish line about a half-mile away and thinking I'd be the third finisher in this race, I heard some of the elite runners approaching. The net result was that Walt finished second, while Pete and I were in the first 10, beating several (incensed) elite runners. The real fun for me, though, was watching Pete each of the three times he was steered back to the course.

In my passage through Taunton I concluded the town's economy must be healthy. The businesses were bulging with customers, there were no empty store fronts, and the streets were crowded with people.

One building in Taunton that left an impression was the Church of Nations Baptist Church, founded in 1837. A two-story edifice with a bell tower, and made of some kind of block stone, it looked like a castle or a fortress.

The folks in these parts are proud of the Taunton Exposition Center that I passed at 12.5 miles into my day. Since it sits a half-mile off the highway, even money could not tempt me, to detour and visit it. I did learn, though, that this is the area's largest show complex and that it's capable of staging any type of entertainment or event.

To the north of Taunton I saw a throwback to the 1940s and 1950s when Angell's Motor Court came into view. Designed like the original motels, it consisted of 40 to 50 units with a car port between each unit. Just can't find any motels like that these days.

In an area that I expected might reek with historical markers, I saw only one. It read, "Anawanrun 1676 historical marker. Site of the capture of Wanpanoag Indian chief Metacomet by Captain Benjamin Church on August 28th, 1676, thus ending King Phillip's War."

A gravel path led to the actual site that was just a few yards off the highway. What the marker omitted was that an Indian traitor lead the British to Phillip's (the name the British gave this Indian chief and by which he is remembered) hiding place and that trying to escape Phillip was killed by an Indian. Another detail omitted, somewhat understandably, is that his head was sent to Plymouth where reportedly it was hung on a pole and remained there for 25 years.

Actually the historical marker I was looking for would have read, "Roger Williams slept here." Seriously, more than once after leaving Plymouth I did wonder if Miles Standish, John Alden, Priscilla Mullens or Roger Williams ever wandered along the area of this road.

Along the way today I went past a motorhome repair shop and, stopping by, I was told they could repair our TV antenna. We limited our day to 16.3 miles to attend to this logistical matter.

Rather relaxing to know that after a little over seven miles tomorrow we would finish Massachusetts.

DAY THREE. On the 17-mile drive to the start of our final day in the state I saw a sign relating to Indians and this strange thought unfolded: How many photos and paintings have I seen of Indian settlements, how many movies have I seen them in, yet in not a one have I seen an outhouse!

Now knuckling down to some basic sociology, what did they do? Unload wherever they got the urge? Or did they have a favorite tree? Oh tell me not in the teepee!

Well, come to think about it, yes, maybe in a teepee – one which, in fact, could have been designed or designated as an outhouse. Weird as all this sounds, it does have a strong scientific connection because how the Indians handled this problem could have a high correlation to the disease rate in their settlements.

Sipping coffee and munching a sweet roll on the way to the start, I sort of felt after being in the same RV park for three successive nights and planning not to return tonight that we were leaving home. Considering that the tab at the Plymouth Rock RV Park was 25 to 30 percent higher than we usually paid, maybe leaving was not all that bad.

Running through the Rehoboth area, I observed that the usual gourmet landmarks – Burger King, KFC, McDonald's – seemed to be prospering, along with some newcomers (at least for us) to the scene, such as Papa Gino.

As I again went past an amusement area – miniature golf, arcade, etc.– I realized that I'd seen one of these about every six miles along this highway. Not quite the frequency of antique shops, though, with 40 to 50 along this highway stretch.

A Model-T driver, passing, honked and waved enthusiastically. I was reminded of the Chevy coupe I had my second year in college, a temperamental vehicle which cost me a total of $90. Barney Pendergast, Joe Quintana and I often ended up pushing the balking Chevy on the way to our college classes.

Passed a place that was, of all things, a combination smoke shop and gun shop. I wanted to name it " The Smoking Gun."

Two sights, one a building, the other a person, impressed me. The Bristol Superior Court Building, made of stone and with a metal roof turned greenish, was remindful of the San Francisco City Hall.

The second sight, one I'd not seen for years in a small city, was a guy hawking newspapers at a street corner. Stirred up memories of my youth when the newsboys would yell, "Extra! Extra!"

The only way to get that sort of action these days is to read Ben Hecht. I hope I'm not slighting Damon Runyon, but I can't remember such in his writings.

Ye gods, how the country has changed was my reaction when I went past a place displaying a eight-by-10 storage shed with a sign on it saying, "Built on your lot for $1800." In time I was carried back to 1937 when my mother rented a two-bedroom home for $35 a month and thought it was too expensive to buy for $3500. Twenty years later it sold for $37,000.

This being Sunday, I held my usual religious services on the road. My first observance here was to note that I am beginning to balk at the word "religion." It seems to smack of being too unionized, too codified, too commercial. But I'm not yet to the point of Alexander Woollcott who said, "To all things cleric, I am allergic."

My focus is more on God . The very minute I say "God," my mind flashes back to when I was running across Arizona and met Denys Savaria, a transcontinental bicyclist. We'd talked a brief while when Denys asked, "Are you close to God? You have to be; you need someone to talk to out here."

I guess Denys' question jolted me because it was so unexpected; rarely do my friends talk about God or religion. I think that they all are God-fearing, but I have no clues as to what most of them believe.

Oh, maybe they voice an opinion on some issue like abortion, but that can be entirely apart from a religious belief (or lack of it). Of all my friends, I'm knowledgeable about the beliefs of only three or so.

One couple believe staunchly in the tenets of their church, and they faithfully follow this church doctrine. Another guy leans toward believing in angels, near-death experiences and out-of-body experiences – subjects on which he is very knowledgeable and well read. A third friend is somewhat of an agnostic.

Maybe because I was not born into the Catholic religion, I find my beliefs fluctuating. While not being born a Catholic, I was baptized into the church as an infant (a neighbor told my mother baptism would improve my sickly health) and had the faith ram-rodded into me all through grammar school and high school while I was a student of the Christian Brothers.

These days I am prone to question some of the church's practices. Confession, for example. Why does a person need an intermediary between him or her and God?

Another example, the church's shabby treatment of women. Why should they be relegated to a status inferior to men? I'm quite sure that many, many women would be better priests than a parade of priests I've endured droning through dull sermons.

Another Church tenet open to questioning: divorce. On the one hand the unequivocal stand that there is absolutely no grounds for divorce, then on the other hand, granting annulments if the petitioner is financially loaded (enter the Kennedys, etc.).

All this mental meandering got me down the road without realizing that the miles were slipping past. When I had about two miles left before reaching the Rhode Island border, I remembered that Elaine had forewarned me she was not making her last regular pit stop. Ever prepared for survival and spotting a donut shop, I got myself a honey-dew donut fix.

Many steps later down the road, I realized a better choice would have been a glazed donut. I was about to retreat, steps be damned, when I realized that the quarter I had left would not buy a glazed donut. So much for survival preparation.

I had just finished savoring my donut when I saw a nursery with this sign, "Celebrate Father's Day by giving him a rose plant." Yikes, whatever happened to a beer, pretzels and a cigar for old dad!

Around two miles I passed through the Seekonk residential area that was barren of any eye-catching sights. The last mile the highway was lined with car dealerships.

Reflecting back on the day's run, it was a leisurely 7.1-mile stroll. There was nothing particularly appealing, but a sufficiency of sights and thoughts to keep me entertained. As with the previous two days no police offers stopped to talk with us, nor did we see any wildlife or snakes. And no dogs chased me. Getting downright dull!

As I approached the Massachusetts/Rhode Island border, my mood was considerably changed from when I was last here – this being when I finished Rhode Island. Then I was a bit uptight, stressed from having been separated from Elaine for three hours and from not knowing where she was at the moment.

Today as I came to the border, I saw her parked nearby. I was as relaxed as a wet noodle.

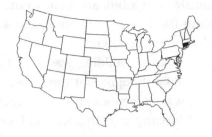

Chapter 15

Connecticut

Not Quite up to Expectations

Dates: *June 9th to 13th, 1997*
Miles: *64.1*
Route: *Start on Highway 7, Massachusetts/Connecticut border, and follow it south to Highway 63. Take 63 south to New Haven and then Highway 10 which leads to water and south Connecticut border.*

DAY ONE. Our first day in Connecticut we frittered away the entire morning scouting different routes – Highways 10, 31 and 16. Rejecting all three as too dangerous (blind corners, too narrow, no bike lane, etc.), we decided to follow the route recommended by Michael D. Taurano of the Connecticut Department of Transportation. His routing began on Highway 7 at the Connecticut/Massachusetts border and followed 7 south to Highway 63 and then stayed on 63 south until reaching the New Haven area and taking Highway 10 to the water.

"This route," Taurano said, "will proceed through the towns of Canaan, Goshen, Litchfield, Waterbury, Naugatuck, and end in New Haven."

Starting in the northwest corner of the state, we were in the hilly part of Connecticut – the Taconic mountain area where our elevation was 2000 feet, only 380 feet short of the state's highest elevation. The good news here, I told myself, was that by the time I reached the water at New Haven, the elevation drop would be close to 2000 feet.

Canaan was the only town on Taurano's list that I saw today. The most impressive building here was Christ Church Episcopal, made of stone and sitting loftily atop a hill. Adjacent to the church itself was an edifice resembling the Tower of London, and adorning it was an ornamental gold clock now defunct.

One intriguing downtown building was the Old Colonial Theater, built in 1923. Sort of old, I thought, but then again a mere child considering that Canaan was incorporated in 1739. Standing beside the theater columns and looking into the arcade, I saw a sign reading, "Temporarily closed due to a death in the family."

Nowhere in town, to my dismay, did I see a bakery or a bookstore. So fie upon you, Canaan; a pox upon your house! (You know, I told myself, that thinking is just silly enough to make me wonder if I've not had too much exposure to the sun and the road!)

A cafe sign, "Hot oven grinders", caught my attention. Just what is an oven grinder? Will have to check that one out before leaving the state.

In town I stopped to study a statue commemorating all the locals who served in World War I. I counted 111 names then re-read the inscription to make sure it said served and not killed or wounded. It did.

In the south end of Canaan I passed by the inescapable Golden Arches that carried a sign, "Hiring, $7 an hour." Higher wage than in California. Could this be a clue to the local economy?

At the junction of Highways 7 and 44 I stopped at Arnold's Garage and made an appointment to get the motorhome serviced (oil change, lube) tomorrow morning. Doing so, I derived some smug satisfaction from knowing I'd score brownie points with Elaine, who had been lobbying to get this work done.

I talked with three people today, other than Elaine. The first conversation was with a guy who drove past me, then turned around to come back and ask, "Do you need a hand?"

"No, but thanks a lot for asking." I felt more inclined to say, "Not a hand, but maybe a blood transfusion, fella."

The second conversation was with a construction worker. I brought up a subject dear to my heart and one of concern hereabouts with all the tall grass I was forced to go through at times when run off the road: "Any poisonous snakes in this area?"

"Not that I know of," he replied.

I didn't carry the resultant complacency very far because in a short distance I stopped to talk with a guy parking a pickup in his driveway. He looked like a guy who spends much time in the outdoors.

I couldn't resist: "Any poisonous snakes in these parts?"

"Oh yeah," he said, "you might see copperheads and you might see rattlers. They killed a rattlesnake down the road last week."

Down with complacency. Up with snake alert!

Caution was the name of the game today. First, the bike lane, only two feet wide, put me close to oncoming cars. Secondly, the road had many "sightless curves," to use the DOT terminology – meaning that a driver approaching me cannot see around the curve and likewise, facing him, I can't see if any vehicle is coming around the corner.

My best course of action, in the name of longevity, is to cross the road and go with traffic where I can then see vehicles in both directions. Luckily traffic was light most of the day, which helped to ease my problems. I also benefited from the 79-degree temperature, the warmest we've had to date this year.

"Deer in the area," the sign read. And a lot of grass, too, I thought. All of which could translate to Lyme disease. Immediate brain response: And remember Lyme disease originated in Lyme, Connecticut.

About seven miles into my day I saw a billboard pointing to a side road and advertising "Music Mountain, America's oldest continuous chamber music festival, started in 1930." Oh the things a man learns on the road!

Despite passing by a number of homes, I did not encounter a dog until eight miles. Rising from his recumbent position, he took a long look at me, then slowly shook his head as if to say, "Too grisly for me," then returned to lying down. The hordes of gnats that had me choking at times were much more troublesome.

Because we got such a late start, we covered only eight miles today. We drove to East Canaan to overnight at the Lone Oaks Campground. There we were learning two things about Connecticut campgrounds: They were primitive, and they were expensive.

I was so absorbed with trying to get a feel for Connecticut today that I did little reminiscing or meditating. I don't know what made me think of it, but I did recall a humorous – and somewhat embarrassing – incident that happened when I was running across the USA, one that only Elaine and I knew about up to this revelation.

Leaving the motorhome just after a pit stop, I was wearing a sweat shirt and sweat pants. As soon as I stepped outside the motorhome, I noticed that the temperature had gone up and the sweats were too warm. Eager to get started, I hurriedly peeled off my sweats and tossed them in the motorhome.

I had gone only 20 yards when I noticed people in a passing car pointing to me and laughing. At the same time I heard Elaine frantically tooting the horn of the motorhome.

I stopped and yelled, "What's the matter?"

"You forget something," she replied.

"What's that?"

"Your shorts!"

Good Lord, I could hardly believe it, but all I had on was my T-shirt and jock strap.

Relaxing last night, I did some reading about Connecticut. One question I had was how did such a small state (third smallest in the country) get such a long name, and what does it mean?

Seems, at least from what I read, it comes from the Algonquin Indian word "Quinnetukut," meaning "place of the long river". The river, in this case, is the Connecticut.

Two tidbits from the night's reading grabbed me. One was that in the Civil War Connecticut had 50,000 volunteers, and 20,000 of them were either killed or missing in action.

The other item was a "blue law" carrying the death penalty for any son who cursed or struck his parents. Left me wondering: Was it ever applied?

Also I read a couple of interesting newspaper articles, both in the *Waterbury Republican American*. The first reported on two guys who were arrested in Kent County for illegally capturing endangered rattlesnakes in the woods near Housantonic River. Which caused me to immediately whip out a map and locate this river, which much to my relief was miles removed from our route.

The second article could be called a human-interest story. It told about the door prize for the winner of a Father's Day drawing at the professional baseball game between the Alley Cats and the River Rats. The prize: a free vasectomy!

DAY TWO. Our usual routine of driving directly to the start and launching the day's run was sabotaged today because the first item on the agenda was having the motorhome serviced at Arnold's Garage. The $54 investment was about $10 over the going rate at home.

While waiting, we took a trip to cholesterol heaven by adjourning to McDonald's next door and consuming Eggs McMuffin. Just to make sure the whole family stayed together, if anything fatal should result from this gastronomy, we splurged by buying a couple of heavenly-bound tickets – er, Egg McMuffins – for Rebel and Brudder.

Once underway I found road conditions similar to yesterday– narrow road, two-foot bike lane, sightless curves, thick forestation, tall grass on each side of the road. Bad but not as bad as the other roads we had scouted. Mercifully semis were rare.

There were three noticeable differences from yesterday: The mosquitoes were out in force, gnats (or some similar insect) stung with more fury, and the hills were steeper and longer. At the first pit stop I doused myself with Avon bath oil, best product I know to repel mosquitoes, and thereafter they were reluctant to use me for a landing pad.

A new problem popped up today when I became aware of flickers radiating from a bone on the inner part of my left knee. It was scary in that the weakness from it caused me to stumble a couple of times.

Years ago I'd been bothered for weeks with a similar problem, but it eventually went away. With it back now, watchful waiting (a phrase President Woodrow Wilson popularized, I vaguely and possibly not accurately recall) would become the name of the game.

Jilted again, I thought, when passing a sign indicating that Cornwall was not on Highway 63 but off to the west. This meant I would miss seeing this town incorporated in 1740.

Working my way up an eight-percent gradient of two miles or more, I entertained several thoughts. Good idea, I mused, that I was heavily sprayed with Avon bath oil because without it, and slowed down as I was on the hill, I'd be mosquito bait.

The next thinking was that being out here is a little like being in a boxing match. Here the idea is to keep moving forward, whether running, jogging or walking. Likewise with boxing, keep moving or get clobbered.

And then came a thought, I knew not why, about the four-star general up for promotion and failing it because he had an affair 12 years prior at a time when he was separated from his wife. Typical stuff in that of all professions the military is held to the most rigid standards, and so held by people who themselves in many cases have sinned worse and gone unpunished.

This is a country where civilian (executive and legislative) abuse of the military has long been a favorite sport. Makes me shudder every time I think how close Harry Truman came in his attempt to abolish the Marine Corps.

My next distraction was the town of Goshen, incorporated in 1739. First thing I noticed on entering the area was the type of rock fence so prevalent in Rhode Island. All the two-story frame homes on the north end of town looked comfortable, roomy and homey.

The three most distinctive sights in town were churches: the somewhat modernistic LDS Church (an outfit about that Dennis Rodman, the illustrated poet laureate of the Chicago Bulls, said uncomplimentary things a few days ago); the Villanova Catholic Church (a two-story building of light colored brick; its adjacent three story rectory looked considerably oversized for a town this small); the Church of Christ Congregational (a two-story frame building with four columns and a bell tower).

My vote for the most impressive building in town went to a two-story mansion atop a hill: at least six bedrooms by my estimate, imposing with an expansive and well-manicured yard. The garage, a detached building of stone, had a Rolls Royce parked in front of it.

Now that's specialization, I thought, while passing by The Angler's and Shooter's Bookstore.

A change of pace in the Goshen area in that for the first time in Connecticut I was out of the hills and into flat agricultural land. The easy going sort of opened up an avenue of day-dreaming.

I thought about my Uncle Paul, a great athlete. I remembered seeing him, at age 45 and wearing bib overalls and high top shoes, high jump 5 feet, 11 inches.

Once, after chopping wood all day, he received a phone call asking if he would substitute for a fighter scheduled to fight the great middleweight champion Stanley Ketchel. Needing the money, Paul agreed.

Ketchel pounded him the first three rounds, at the end of which the announcer told the crowd that Paul, after working all day cutting wood, substituted at the last moment. The crowd then rallied to his support, and he held Ketchel to a draw the rest of the fight.

Thought about Joe Quintana, now dead, with whom I played on four different basketball teams and who, while at the University of California, Berkeley, shared an apartment with me (if a kitchen and bedroom with a community bath down the hall can be called an "apartment"). Because Joe had worked at a cannery and was thus able to purchase cans of food for five cents each, our kitchen was well stocked.

These cans had no labels, just coded cannery numbers. When Joe had to quit Cal because of his father's illness, I was left with a kitchen full of canned products identified only by code numbers that I didn't know. At least I could identify the catsup, all 24 bottles, which did have labels.

Thought about Paul McAvoy, a talented 19-year old-who was in my intelligence section in the 21st Marines. After Bougainville when we returned to Guadalcanal, I was transferred to the north end of the island, apart from the 21st Marines.

One day Mac hitched a ride from the south end of the island to visit me. Since he was wearing corporal stripes, I could not take him to the officers' mess for lunch in that uniform. I gave him a shirt of mine, one without any insignia, to wear and then took him to lunch in the mess.

We got away with it and the experience made Mac's day. Least I could do for a kid who cared enough to visit me.

Coming out of the nine-mile pit stop, I almost had to flog myself to get going. It was that kind of a day.

The knee kept sending distress signals. The sultry, 85-degree heat was getting to me because this was only the second warm day of this year's outing, and my energy seemed at low ebb.

A bit of a diversion when I saw what looked like a resort, a sprawling, white two-story frame building, hotel size. The sign read, "Connecticut Junior Republic, Founded 1924."

Now what's that all about? Curious, I wandered inside to ask a couple of questions, not quite sure what to expect. It turned out to be a facility for emotionally disturbed male adolescents. Subsequently I learned that Andy Bisset, a Marine Corps classmate, is on the Republic's Board of Governors.

Elaine was surprised today when she was parked at the last pit stop and some teenagers on bikes, having seen me, stopped to ask her, "Is that the old man who ran across United States?" How'd they know that? The best we could figure out was that they got this info from watching a Health Rider infomercial in which I appeared with other ancient athletes.

Shortly after I left the Junior Republic, a couple of college girls stopped to ask if I knew where Bush Lane was. "It's a place where they repair Volkswagens," they said.

When they told me it was in Goshen, I informed them they had a few miles to go to reach that town. Ye gods, I thought, in college and they don't have sense enough to use a map. Oh what the hell, more adventurous their way!

Our running day, which began at 11:30 A.M., ended after 14.6 miles, placing us at the northern edge of Litchfield. As we drove to the RV park, I found myself hoping that tomorrow would reveal some of the New England charm that had eluded me so far.

DAY THREE. This day was unusual for me because for the first time in this state I started in T-shirt and running shorts – a yellow shirt with "Running Across All 50 States" printed on the front of it and red shorts. Despite my flashy colors and antiquity I attracted no attention as I jogged through town. My brief attire was understandable since the weather prediction was 95 degrees.

From the very moment I began to edge into Litchfield, and while going past some stately and luxurious homes, I became aware that here I would be tasting the flavor of New England. So attractive were some of the homes that I felt compelled to stop and photograph them, knowing I would have no earthly use for the photos. One three-story home dated back to 1760.

As I stood in the town square and looked around, I seemed to sense an air of serenity and dignity emanating from this town dating back to 1719. I tried but failed to visualize the village as it was back in 1790 when it was the third-largest city in the United States, surpassed only by New York and Philadelphia.

Then it was 2-1/2 times larger than its present population of 8400. The green itself, which dates back to 1770, was certainly part of the scene then.

In today's world Litchfield has things going in all directions. Just last weekend 1300 runners lined up here for a race. The Litchfield Jazz Festival, held annually in August, is a hot newcomer to the jazz scene.

The Litchfield hills area abounds with antique stores, art galleries, superior lodging in inns, resorts, and bed and breakfast houses, with museums, with a variety of shops, with theater attractions and with renowned restaurants. I got the impression that you'd better bring a satchel of money if you plan to recreate in these parts very long. The elegance is here and with the prices to match it.

I did not linger to explore any of the stores whose addresses are listed as being On-the-Green. As I worked my way out of town, I found the south exit a duplicate of my north entrance in that it was a street lined with trees and stately homes, any of which 99 percent of Americans could look at and say, "I wish I had a pad like that!" I couldn't help but wonder, Where does all this money come from?

When I went past the William Marsh home, dating back to 1761, I again whipped out my Olympus to record it on film. My God, another home more than 200 years old. Makes me, only 80, feel like a kid!

A short distance out of town I stopped to talk with a state trooper. From him I learned that there are approximately 950 troopers in the state patrol.

That seemed well-stocked to me considering Connecticut has only three million residents and is the third-smallest state geographically. By comparison, if I remember correctly, both Montana and Wyoming have only about 180 troopers each, and they are the ninth- and fourth-largest states, respectively, albeit their populations are about one-third and one-sixth that of Connecticut.

The trooper confirmed my previous observation that the state's patrol cars are of different colors. "Their only identification," he said, "is the roof rack."

When I pulled out my cassette recorder to make notes, he got jumpy and asked, "What's that for?" I had to explain what I was doing.

Much of the day the narrow road, without a running shoulder and with many curves and heavy traffic, put a damper on my enjoyment. In a few spots, as when I ascended hills, the road was so narrow and curvy I had to get outside the guard rail and walk. I kept telling myself, Focus on survival and not speed.

To take my mind off my troubles, I deliberately concentrated on disassociating, and doing so I entertained a potpourri of thoughts. Got a laugh when I thought back to World War II and George Stone Saussy, a South Carolina native and fellow air scout, whom we fondly called "Sharecropper."

Sometimes we were transferred from one carrier to another via a destroyer using a Jacob's Ladder, a contraption that looked like an oversized basket and was suspended on a rope running between the two ships. On one such transfer George's parachute bag containing, among other things, six bottles of bourbon and a Confederate flag, bounced out of the basket and into the ocean.

"I'll make the damn Yankees pay," George said, and he filed a claim against the government. The humorous part was the government actually paid the claim.

A variety of other thoughts continued to tumble through my mind before I zoomed in on three hectic months of my life in 1941 when at Quantico, Virginia, I was in training to become a Marine Corps officer. They called us "officer candidates."

They paid us $21 a month, most of which, out of necessity, went for laundry, toilet articles and cleaning materials for our Marine Corps gear. They kept us fully occupied from 5:30 A.M. to 10 P.M. while putting us to all sorts of tests.

Almost daily someone was dismissed. I saw a guy succumb to pressure and say to a superior, "To hell with it. You can shove it up to where the sun doesn't shine!" For him that was good-bye.

If it was discovered that a guy was married, he was sent packing. One morning during our cleaning chores, a guy, rushed for time as we always were, rinsed his mop in a nearby drinking fountain instead of going down the hall to the proper basin. He was dismissed for poor judgment.

At the junction of Highway 63 and 109 when I saw a lady setting up a portable hot dog stand, evidently a daily ritual for her, I wanted to yell, "Watch out, lady, McDonald's is looking over your shoulder." Wouldn't surprise me a bit to learn that McDonald's had done a market survey of the location.

When I came into the 13-mile pit stop , Elaine tormented me by saying, "It's only 68 degrees in here, but it's 94 out on the road."

The part of Waterbury that I passed through was a tough transit for me – mainly because of heavy traffic, stop lights and being confined to sidewalks. I did stop to gawk at a couple of old homes both dating back to the late 1760s.

Little else caught my attention. Maybe I was just getting tired and concerned with finishing.

The lasting memory I took from the Waterbury area was of a cemetery and a grave that contained the remains of 29 Revolutionary War soldiers killed in 1776. Eleven of them were officers.

Going past some car dealerships, I saw three American flags flying. Reminded me of the recent events of flag burning and the ACLU defense of such. Wonder how the ACLU would react if some of its offices were burned? Tempt me not, Satan!

By the time we reached 16.3 miles, I was more than ready to quit even though I felt like a wimp when thinking back to my 26 miles days when running across the USA.

This had been a somewhat stressful day. I'd expended considerable effort, I'd not had any lively experiences, and the heat was oppressive.

We had only a 12 mile drive to the nearest RV park. But once again Connecticut failed us.

The place had only 20 amp electrical hooks, insufficient to run our air conditioner. Another night in a hot motorhome. Hardly conducive to R&R, and rapidly becoming the number-one problem in this state.

I feel that two of the keys to my success are good food and sufficient sleep. Elaine's food offerings exceed what is needed but Connecticut's inadequate RV parks are depriving me of sleep.

DAY FOUR. Starting this morning, I felt a certain amount of buoyancy from knowing that if I covered about 17 miles today I'd have only seven or so tomorrow and Connecticut, my 42nd state, would be a fiat accompli. Except for the Litchfield area and some stately homes Connecticut has turned out to be devoid of the New England charm I had expected, and difficult mainly because of the running conditions. And yet, judging from the reconnaissances we had made, these running conditions were as good as they get in Connecticut.

Just why wasn't Connecticut fusing enthusiasm in me, I had asked myself several times. I surmised that from the glowing reports I'd received about New England, I was expecting to step into an enchanting environment, one sort of like I'd seen in the Litchfield area and nowhere else.

Maybe the problem was that I was just expecting too much from New England. And on that score the jury was still out: I had yet to run Maine, Vermont and New Hampshire.

By now I was tired of waiting roadside for cars to pass, tired of retreating to the tall grass to avoid cars, tired of sometimes having to jump the guard rail to escape an oncoming car. I decided to live dangerously today by clinging to the 14-inch bike lane, to keep moving cautiously in it and to ignore the cars roaring towards me at 55 miles per hour.

A bit hairy-scary. At least, so I consoled myself, my yellow T-shirt and red shorts made me easy to see.

Early in the going, and unexpectedly, I faced a traffic monster at the junctions of Highways 63 and 64. It looked like a scene out of Paris traffic, cars maneuvering in all directions.

For five minutes I waited for an opening; then, seeing none, in desperation I threw my arms wildly about to attract attention, slowly jogged across the road and found myself smothered with surprise after negotiating a safe passage. But what the hell, Russian roulette isn't always fatal!

I had hoped to get a peek at the town of Middlebury, but a sign at the junction of Highway 188 told me the town was off to the west. As close as I came was to Middlebury Crossroads Shopping Center housing Mabel's Restaurant, Gooey Donuts and Middlebury Medical Center.

Shortly afterward, and for the first time on Highway 63, I spotted a sign pointing to New Haven. Very encouraging.

Coming upon a Middlebury police officer whose vehicle was concealed by bushes, I stopped for a brief conversation. The talk was brief because his body language told me he wanted to concentrate on his radar.

He confirmed my estimates on the distance to New Haven and the water, our finish. "I like it a lot better here in the winter," he told me. "Fewer people, and it's really beautiful with the snow on the ground."

Three times today three different old biddies, each driving a Cadillac, raised the fur on my back – especially the one coming toward me as I rounded a corner. Two of them were driving with their cars occupying half the bike lane and the other fully occupied it.

By the time I encountered the third one, I lost my cool, planted myself on the fog line and stood there, my body language radiating, Hit me if you dare! Seeing me, she immediately turned into the slow lane, and as she did I thought, How lucky nobody was behind you because you certainly didn't look to see if it was clear.

I did not behave as recklessly whenever a local truck driver (bakery, produce, etc.) approached me because by now I've learned to watch out for these guys when near a city. Uniformly they are reluctant to give me even an iota of running space.

Despite my determination to stay planted in the bike lane and run there, in the course of the day I had to jump the guard rail a few times to avoid fast-approaching cars. Seemed that some drivers in these parts were possessive of their proprietary domain. Such were my woes on the road today.

By way of contrast, Elaine said she found most of the Connecticut drivers to be courteous, though some seemed to be fond of tailgating.

Here I am getting close to finishing another state, I told myself, and I should be enjoying the satisfaction of that but, instead I'm focused on not getting hit by a car. Well, that's a bit understandable because, after all, life is beautiful

Going through the Nagatuck area was a considerable improvement and more relaxing because I had the protection of a sidewalk. I didn't see the downtown section of Nagatuck, which Highway 63 misses by about three blocks. Gasoline, priced at $1.50 a gallon compared to the $1.09 we'd paid in some states, gave me a feel for the local economy.

When I came to the junction of Highways 63 and 68, I took notice of one of Connecticut's covered bridges. The setting I saw in the Nagatuck area was pleasant – beautiful trees and a small stream paralleling the roads, modest and well-kept homes, and a neatly maintained city park. My guess was that most of the residents work in nearby Waterbury. But not the dentists; I passed the offices of six different dentists.

Leaving the Nagatuck area, I crossed a bridge over a river and a railroad, and atop the bridge I turned around to look in the direction of downtown Nagatuck. All I could see was a town nestled in a heavy tree setting, above which rose four steeples (I judged three of them to be from churches and one from the city hall) and a huge manufacturing plant.

A roadside sandwich shop advertised grinders. Ah, my big chance to find out about grinders. What I learned was that a grinder is nothing more than a sub sandwich, or so the informant told me.

Just past Nagatuck I went by the Peter Paul Candy Company. So this is the birthplace of all those Almond Joy candy bars I've devoured over the years.

In another mile I passed a construction site for a new Wal Mart. The amount of excavation going on was unbelievable; appeared an entire mountain was being transformed, and it appeared to be a project costing over a million dollars. Traffic is already congested on this road; Wal Mart will bring it to a standstill.

Elaine was parked for the 12-mile pit stop in front of a veterinary office. Before I could say anything, she said, "Don't worry. I got permission to park here.

"Asking for it was sort of fun. First I told them that I am pit crewing for my husband who's running across the state, and they could barely believe anyone would run in this humid weather. Then when they're still weighing that, I deliver the punch line by adding, 'And he's 80 years old!' "

A while later when I saw the Daries Beecher home – a two-story white frame building dating back to 1807 – I wondered if the owner were any relation to Harriet Beecher Stowe. Seemed possible, even likely, since she was born in nearby Litchfield, as I learned while passing through that town.

Going through the Bethany area, all I saw was peewee-sized post office, a Citgo Gas Station, and the Bethany Episcopal Church founded in 1799.

We were about a quarter-mile north of the junction of Highways 63 an 114 when we finished our 17.2-mile day.

Time after time today my thoughts reverted to my grandfather, my mother's father and the only grandparent with whom I ever came into contact. And I did not become aware of him until my junior high school days when, for the first time in our lives, we were both in the same place. That place was the home of his son, my Uncle Paul, a place where I spent a couple of weeks each summer working around the ranch and picking fruit.

My grandfather, Julian Hontou, lived in a small cabin about 40 yards from Paul's house, and about the cabin was where he spent most of his day. Sometimes, though, I would see him at breakfast, a meal where his menu never varied.

He took three pieces of bread, tore them into bitesized pieces, and put them in a soup bowl. He sprinkled sugar on the bread, then filled the bowl with coffee laced with milk. As I understood it, this breakfast was a carryover from his native France from which he had emigrated.

Another thing that never varied was his attire: a wide-brimmed felt hat with the crown flattened circularly, bib overalls, a blue work shirt, a heavy belt around his waist and high-top shoes. He was covered with foliage – a full head of hair and a full beard, both a dark gray.

From what I saw, he was a loner and a man I judged to have lived a sad life – mainly as a result of his young wife, whom he'd brought from France. She had drowned when my mother, the youngest of his three children, was only three years old. He was left to forge a living for his two sons and a daughter and to care for them.

About the closest he and I came to conversation was to exchange morning greetings. I'm not quite sure why we didn't talk, possibly because he was accustomed to being alone.

For sure I was blind to what a wealth of information I could have gleaned from him about our family background, about which I knew practically nothing. As a kid I did not have the poise to approach him. If I had been thinking, maybe I could have persuaded him to teach me French.

In retrospect I regret that I did not at least try to get to know him. How many other kids, I wondered, are making a similar mistake today?

DAY FIVE. The core idea today was to cover the remaining seven or so miles in Connecticut with whatever rapidity I could muster, then to fire up the motorhome and head for Vermont. That made it much of a business day – no lolly-gagging along the way, no detouring into a donut shop, no browsing in a bookstore, no stopping to read historical markers, certainly no memorial services for fallen roadkill and no jaunting into cemeteries to read tombstone markers, just onward Christian soldier!

I started by doing something I rarely do, running with traffic. The reason for that was simple. The bike lane with traffic was twice as wide as the one against traffic.

Nonetheless for me it is always an eerie feeling to hear the traffic creeping up my back. On that score I've got to hand it to the bicyclists. They literally put their lives in the hands of drivers.

I'd gone only 1.4 miles, all of it in a misty rain, before I was into a built-up area, store fronts and all such, which along with heavy traffic continued the rest of the day. Traffic density and the 55-MPH speed limit made street crossings difficult, but my high visibility (yellow shirt, red shorts) and lightning speed helped to alleviate that problem.

Around two miles I negotiated the I-15 underpass and emerging from it came upon a sidewalk. For the remainder of today's miles I had the protection of a sidewalk, and the only danger I faced was when crossing streets and dodging the fast traffic.

The sights along the way were varied. Not too long after passing through a tacky residential area, garbage strewn all about the sidewalk, I came to a trendy area replete with coffee houses, craft shops and jewelry stores. On some street corners vendors were hawking newspapers, something I've not seen on the West Coast in recent years.

I went past two city parks, two miles apart at most, and was puzzled as to why one was neatly maintained and the other looked abandoned. Seeing a Holocaust memorial designed to commemorate each of the camps was a new experience for me.

When I arrived at Boulevard Street and turned right to follow Highway 10, I thought about the confusion this street caused me last night when I was studying the map. I kept looking for the name of the boulevard until I finally realized the name was Boulevard Street.

Remembering Providence, Rhode Island, and our getting separated there, Elaine and I studied the map last night. We were locked into the same route today, leaving nothing to chance. The password was no more Providence fiascoes.

Going along, I happened to look to my right and what did my

eyes behold but the Yale Bowl, scene of the university's football games. Let's hear it for the bulldogs, I felt like yelling, but I restrained myself because I was not sure bulldogs was the correct name of the Yale mascot.

In fact, I wasn't even sure of why or how the name bulldogs popped into my head. From what I saw, there seemed to be an abundance of unused, empty land in the vicinity of the bowl, a half-mile of nothing but weeds and trees.

Hundreds of seagulls were patrolling three of the university's soccer fields. I did not see Jonathan among them.

An unexpected sight when I saw a deer entrapped in a cyclone fence. I had to take a second look to make sure it was dead. What a horrible death it must have suffered, entrapped there and starving.

The fence was but three feet from the sidewalk and 10 from the street. Many people must have seen the deer. Why didn't someone initiate a rescue effort?

At our last pit stop Elaine reported that while listening to the truck drivers on their CB's, she heard them refer to me as "Lightfoot." Ah c'mon, fellas, I wasn't really that slow!

Speaking of Elaine, she hit a new high today in jockeying the motorhome. Near the end of the day she found herself on the Highway 95 approach, realized this was a mistake and made a U-turn while still on the approach ramp.

Her story: No cars were coming in either direction, and she considered the move safe. But she did grant she had to expedite the maneuver. She justified herself by saying, "I didn't want us to get separated like we did in Providence."

Our finish, after a 7.5-mile day, was in the water not far from the City Point Yacht Club. Somewhat a refreshing change to have a distinctive state boundary, the water, instead of the usual nondescript spot, indicated only by a state boundary sign that marked most of our recent state finishes.

After finishing, we stayed around only long enough to devour a couple of sub sandwiches. The next move was to head for Vermont where, after 138 miles of driving, we arrived at Hidden Acres Campground.

I was looking forward to retiring early because I didn't get much sleep last night. That was understandable because we stayed in a town named Clinton and, even worse yet, at the Clinton RV Park. This Clintonese made me ill at ease, disturbing my sleep.*

We decided that our first action tomorrow would be to check out our planned Vermont route and see if it was safe for Elaine's driving and my running. We knew it was hilly and curvy, but the question needing an answer: Was it something we could handle?

In making this feasibility check, we knew it had to be quite bad for us to reject it because we operated somewhat along the lines of the Marine Corps recruiting poster which read, "We didn't promise you a rose garden."

---

* The remarks about President Clinton that I make in this book were written months before the Starr Report and do not stem from it. Rather they stem from the fact that in time of war Clinton dodged the draft, and while subsidized by the government on a Rhodes scholarship he demonstrated against his country and the military at a time when some of my good friends in the Marine Corps were being killed in combat.

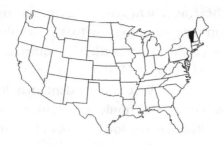

Chapter 16

Vermont

Green Mountains, Twisty Roads and Maple Syrup

Dates: *June 14th to 16th, 1997*
Miles: *48.3*
Route: *Start on Highway 9, New York/Vermont border, and follow 9 east to Brattleboro and Connecticut River, New Hampshire border.*

DAY ONE. No doubt about it, looking at a map of Vermont we decided the two best routes across the state were both east-west – Highway 4 in the center of the state going through Rutland and Woodstock, and in the southern part of the state Highway 9 from Bennington to Brattleboro.

I asked Mike Scelsi, a Marine Corps classmate and resident of Manchester, Vermont, for help in evaluating these routes. Mike talked this over with his friend Jim Hand, a fellow Vermont resident, and both agreed that Highway 9 was the preferable route.

John Taylor of the Vermont Department of Transportation told me that Route 9 was the shorter route but also a mountainous and twisty road. Route 4, he said, has better shoulders, a higher traffic flow and "the great villages of Castleton and Woodstock."

He suggested that if we were leaning toward Highway 9, it would be a good idea to drive it first. And that we did by driving east to west from Brattleboro to Bennington.

Doing so, we got off to an early start, being on the road shortly after five A.M., because Rebel and Brudder rousted us from sleep. Seems that around four o'clock some squirrels started cavorting around the motorhome.

Seeing and hearing them, the dogs went bananas, charging around the motorhome jumping up to the windows, barking and whining. Not being able to persuade the squirrels to vamoose, the only way Elaine and I could quell the dogs was to flee the RV park.

As we drove Highway 9, it was evident that John Taylor was a master of understatement. He should have said very mountainous and extremely twisty. Although we found 9 marginal, we decided to go with it because it was the shortest route across the state and it was scenic.

About halfway across the state, I told Elaine, "Vermont is certainly aptly named." I was referring to it being named after its evergreen mountains. The name comes from the French words "vert," meaning green, and "mont," meaning mountains.

The Vermont/New York border on Highway 9, our starting spot, was marked only by a boundary sign, no geographical landmarks. After we followed our ritual of taking the usual start-boundary photos, I ran eastward well aware that, with mountains and a twisty road the villains, I'd have some tough sledding for three days.

Forget that and enjoy this, I told myself as I relished the luxury of a three-foot shoulder on the 1.5-mile jog into Bennington.

I'd read about Vermont farming and dairying (supplying much of New England, including Boston) and environmentalists, so it was not much of a surprise to pass a prosperous-looking farm nor to see that the road signs were of a woodsy design instead of the usual green and white metal type.

Was a bit of a surprise, though, to see that the price of Vermont maple syrup was $28 a gallon. I soon found out that I could not go a mile without seeing maple syrup advertised for sale.

At one corner in west Bennington five crosses marking the scene of a fatal accident in 1996 caught my attention. My guess: The driver took the curve, which has a sharp drop-off, too fast.

I was awed by the beauty, almost majestic, of some stately two-story homes, all of vintage, along two blocks on the west edge of town. Sort of tragic, I decided, that the beauty of this scene was flawed by the heavy flow of highway traffic.

It resembles the campanile of the University of California, Berkeley, was my first thought when I saw the Bennington Memorial. At 306 feet high it was the tallest battle monument in the world when completed in 1891, and it commemorates the Battle of Bennington when American general John Stark defeated the expeditionary forces of British general John Burgoyne.

"Devoted to the art of the animal kingdom," so read the sign on a gallery I passed. Why did that trigger thoughts of bison being slaughtered in Yellowstone National Park and of exterminators hired to kill deer in Connecticut?

Now there's a place that will quickly separate a tourist from his money, was my reading on seeing Camelot Village, consisting of several craft shops. Before going in there, it might be a good idea to stop at Joseph Cerniglia Winery across the street, belt down a couple of drinks and thus be able to absorb the sticker shock of prices.

The Four Chimneys Inn–"Elegance in lodging and dining", said the sign – and even on a passing glance, that was the feeling I was left with: elegance. Dinner and a night there would result in a vigorous massage for anyone's Visa card.

I felt downright guilty in not stopping when going by the photogenic Old First Church (usual New England needle-sharp white church spire), built in 1806, and in not wandering into the adjacent cemetery to locate the grave of Robert Frost whose poems I've always enjoyed. His self-written epitaph, "I had a lover's quarrel with life."

Would also have liked to stop at the Bennington Museum and seen the collection of Grandma Moses' paintings.

That's the place I'd like to be if a tornado hits this area now, I told myself, while looking at the Sacred Heart St. Francis Desles Church, made of granite.

Look around and enjoy this, I again reminded myself as I came into the business section of Bennington, a flat area where I was protected by a sidewalk – the easiest running I'd have across the state. That thought on my mind, I heard a young guy asking, "Are you really doing that?" He was referring to my T-shirt, "Running Across All 50 States."

We stood on the sidewalk for a brief conversation. He said his name was Tom Warmin, that he was a dietitian at the local hospital.

"I'm also an avid hiker, skier and bicyclist," he volunteered. "Not enough snow to ski here. The closest place is Prospect Mountain, 10 miles to the west. They'd probably let you park your motorhome on their lot."

Two blocks later I realized I'd missed an opportunity to catch up on some local history. I should have asked Tom if the Catamount Tavern, where General Stark organized his Green Mountain Boys, still exists.

The array of motels, hotels, inns and restaurants was evidence of Bennington being a tourist mecca. It took me a while to decipher what was different here from many other small towns, then it dawned: Everything here (lodging, restaurants, shops) reflected a touch of class. Nothing tacky did I see.

The most amusing sight today was a guy riding a tractor mower followed by his three Boxers. Crossing a downtown street and lined up in tandem, they looked like soldiers on parade.

The three blocks or so of business section was bustling with activity, people shopping, sidewalk cafes, tourists walking and gawking.

Arriving at our first pit stop, I had to admit that Elaine is displaying more expertise in selecting pit-stop sites. This one was across the street from Dunkin Donuts, beside a bookstore and a block from the post office where we had mail to deposit.

In this town of 16,000 the only luxury homes I saw were the stately mansions as we entered the built-up area. The rest were modest frame homes.

On the east side of town, and somewhat unexpectedly – after all, Vermont is sometimes referred to as quintessential New England – many of the homes were rundown and in need of paint, and the yards were untidy.

As I exited town and was plunged into dangerous running conditions (nine-inch bike lane, narrow road, sightless curves), I regretted not being able to take time out to visit Bennington College. Katherine Kiefer – one of its graduates, a runner and practicing attorney – had given me good reports on it.

Once out of town and until the end of our day, limited to 13 miles because of a late start after our reconnaissance, I operated on red alert while avoiding the many cars on the road. Actually there were as many motorcycles as cars, but they posed considerably less danger.

Well, at least I won't have to ask the natives if there are any snakes around here. This was my reaction as I stepped over a dead snake.

Engulfed with greenery and mountains, I thought back to Connecticut where the setting was often similar. The difference here was that for some reason Vermont was more woodsy. Definitely, Connecticut had more industrial pollution. And, yes, Vermont carries this greenery to the fullest with car license plates being that color.

After Bennington the only settlement I went through was Woodward – a hamlet of 321 people, some modest homes, all about 100 yards apart, and a town meeting house chartered in 1753.

One of our reasons besides time of day for our stopping precisely at 13 miles was that put us at the location of Greenwood Lodge. It advertised campsites, all of which turned out to be a unique experience because the "sites" consisted of parking the motorhome within three feet of the lodge building and parallel to it, then hooking up to electrical and water connections attached to the lodge.

Sort of an odd scene with six motorhomes attached to the lodge. But these were the only 30-amp hookups available between Bennington and Brattleboro, a convenience we much appreciated. And in these surroundings we spent a quiet night between the Taconic Mountains and the Green Mountains to the south.

Damn it, I told myself several times today, I wish I had the safety of a three- to four-foot bike lane so that I could study and absorb some of the superlative scenery surrounding me instead of having to be constantly alert in order to avoid getting embraced by a car. Only going through Bennington could I safely look around without endangering myself.

At one point today, and for no particular reason, I thought back on some of the firsts in my life. Like the first time I ever shot a deer, and this was at age 12. Now, 68 years later, I can still hear his "bah" as, back broken and dying, he rolled down a hill into a gully.

I also thought about the first time, this was around age 11, when in company with some cronies, I invaded Piggly Wiggly, the first self-serve market in Sacramento. Each of us stashed three candy bars under our sweaters and, trying our best to look innocent, exited. The pickings are too easy, we decided; self-serve markets won't last long!

Then my mind wandered to the first time I climbed into a torpedo bomber (also known as a TBF or TBM, depending on the manufacturer, Grumman or Martin) and felt as if the climb was six stories high. In less than a week, a veteran by now, it seemed only one step up.

Then I recalled the first time I soloed an airplane and, once aloft, I couldn't understand why the thing was so thunderously noisy until

I looked at my RPM setting and saw it was almost redline.

There was also the exaltation of the first time I landed a permanent job – this as a teacher in Sacramento, 1940, annual salary $1548, after five years of college and a master's degree. In those days that $129 a month seemed big.

I reflected on completing our first run across any state – California in 1990, 260 miles – and the jubilation Elaine and I felt over this accomplishment and the confidence it inspired. Little did we realize what would follow.

Now I'm wondering: What will follow the next two days and 35 miles in Vermont?.

DAY TWO. Waking up and turning on the coffee pot, I heard Elaine say, "Happy Father's Day." As she handed me a present and a card, I thought, Damn lucky guy to have somebody who cares so much. Good Lord, she even remembers the Marine Corps birthday!

The temperature outside registering 30 degrees dampened my enthusiasm for getting on the road. Old bones don't take kindly to cold weather.

When we started at 7:40 A.M., the temperature was still under 40. To make matters worse, I discovered, half a mile down the road, that my water bottle had sprung a leak and my shorts and wind pants were soaked. Not only uncomfortably cold but sort of embarrassing because, seeing me, some drivers would conclude the old man has an incontinence problem.

Fresh in my mind as I started were a couple of things about Vermont I'd learned last night when reading a pamphlet in the lodge. Vermont ranks 49th among states in population (barely over half a million) and 43rd in land size. Its biggest city, Burlington, has only 40,000 residents.

But Vermont claims to rank first in the independence of its people – an independence dating all the way back to 1777 when it became an independent republic and stayed that way until 1791 when it was admitted as the 14th state in the Union. I also learned it's unique in being the only New England state without a coastline; no broiled lobster or clam bakes here!

In the early miles a potpourri of observations and thoughts occupied me. The idiot in the sports car speeding past at 65 miles per hour worried me – not that he might get killed or injured, but that he might hit someone along the way, even Elaine parked at a pit stop.

Going through an area filled with water, trees protruding from it, was remindful of similar areas in Alaska where we saw moose. Maybe I should be on moose alert.

Seeing a Woodford State Park sign, I again lamented the fact that Vermont state parks don't have electrical hookups.

Charging up hills, I began to question the direction I'd chosen for this route. Maybe if I were going east-west instead of west-east, I'd have more downhill. Oddly, contrary to my usual procedure, I had not given elevation gain/decline any thought when choosing the direction we'd run in Vermont.

Elaine and I both got a laugh out of what Vermont dubs a "rest area," consisting solely of a turnout and a place to park. Quite a comedown from the typical state rest area that has restrooms, ample parking, vending machines and tourist information.

You're either very dumb or very courageous, I thought, as I saw two bicyclists head west on this road. Hard to imagine the scenario when these guys round a sightless curve and a speeding car, not aware of them, descends on them from the rear.

Embraced by the forested mountains, warmed by the sun, feeling unusually vibrant and healthy, I heard myself saying aloud, "Thank you, God, for this at age 80!"

My Deo gratias was a reminder to practice my usual Sunday on the road ritual of observing the Sabbath. Doing so, I asked myself: Am I, like Philip Nolan who became a man without a country, becoming a man without a religion? Well, to be sure, I'm not on the team as a practicing Catholic. Actually by their rules I am ineligible because of marrying a divorced woman. What the hell has that got to do with what kind of a person I am? As for the divorced woman, compared to me, she's saintly.

Oddly, though, when I attend church – as I quite often do just to be in a house of prayer and to lobby my cause before the Supreme Executive Officer – I attend a Catholic church. Once there and exposed to all the singing and ecumenical liturgy, I have to look around and to make sure I am in a Catholic church. This is not the quiet prayer setting of the church in which I was raised. But these days, looking around, I am 90 percent sure of being in a Catholic church when I listen to the sermon (called a "homily" these days) and it's dull, uninspiring and trite – par for 90 percent of Catholic priests these days. I feel like a stranger in my own church.

Sort of got carried away, didn't you, I told myself when reviewing all those thoughts. And up came the question: Having so spoken, so confessed, stand I now on the threshold of excommunication?

At least I have a long way to go before I catch up with Thomas Paine, who said, "I do not believe in the creed professed by the Jewish church, by the Roman church, by the Greek church, by the Turkish church, by the Protestant church, nor by any church that I know of. My own mind is my own church."

Tough as running conditions were today, I was grateful to see no semis on the road. I was dodging cars so often that I felt like a matador.

This was not one of those days of simply putting one foot in front of the other and moving forward. Instead – fighting a twisty, mountainous road, sightless curves, and no running space – I walked a tightrope. For me it was general quarters all day.

On today's 17.9-mile journey I went through two settlements. The first one, Salisbury, consisted of nothing but four homes located roadside. No distractions here.

Wilmington, a town of 2000 inhabitants, provided entertainment for about one mile. Sort of a surprise to see the Green Mountain Flagship Company boat docked on a small lake.

Hoping to find a book to add to my library of running books, I ducked into a rare book store on what turned out to be an unsuccessful hunting expedition. I also took time out to study some of the superb craftsmanship in John Meleodit's woodwork shop.

This Sunday downtown Wilmington was 42nd and Broadway – people crowding the streets, the shops, the restaurants, the sidewalk cafes. I noted three typical Vermont inns: the Vermont House Tavern and Restaurant, a three-story building with four columns in front and dating back to the early 1900s by my estimate; across the street, the Cross Inn, also three stories with a porch around most of the first floor; and, my favorite, the White House Inn, sitting on a hill about one mile east of town, a sprawling two-story frame building reeking of ancestry and of good taste.

The name of a cemetery one mile east of downtown unsettled me: Restland. Just rubbed me the wrong way.

However, in a couple of miles I felt better about Vermont cemeteries when I went past the best-maintained cemetery I've seen in all our travels so far this year.

Had a fleeting flashback today to 1942 when Bob Spangler, Bill Stephens and I were newly commissioned second lieutenants being transferred from Quantico, Virginia, to California. We decided that we'd make the trip on United Airlines.

The plane was a DC-3 and the coast-to-coast flight, with several letdowns, took 18 hours, which wasn't too bad since this was a sleeper flight. In fact, it had its moments because safety regulations required that each of the passengers be strapped in his berth during takeoffs and landings, and the flight stewardess peeked into each berth during landings and takeoffs to make sure the belt was fastened. Nice to have a comely stewardess (and they were much so in those days!) fussing over you in the middle of the night!

I still have a vivid memory of the dinner service on that flight – china, linen, a flower for each table, and a full menu of soup, salad, entree, vegetable, potatoes, dessert and drink. All back in the days when the pilots earned $3000 a year.

Our finish provided the most spectacular sight of the day: Hogsback Mountain where, from the balcony of a gift shop or from the 100-Mile Restaurant, the setting offered a view of 100 miles across green mountains. After Elaine and I had admired it for a while, I photographed it even though I knew full well the photo could not do this breathtaking scene justice.

After finishing, we had to make a choice of where to overnight. We had three alternatives: drive 22 miles east over the mountain roads to Brattleboro to a conventional RV park with hookups; drive 18 miles back west over the hills to Greenwood Lodge where we were last night; drive 1.5 miles to Molly Stark State Park, which had no electrical hookups but where we could run our generator during daylight hours.

For Elaine, who'd had her fill of driving the twisty mountainous road, the decision was easy: Molly Stark.

DAY THREE. Camping in Molly Stark State Park last night was, on the one hand, luxury compared to accommodations we often had when going across the USA and simply overnighting at some roadside spot.

On the other hand, Molly Stark was primitive compared to being in an RV park and having full electrical, water and sewer hookups.

On the plus side the park's 23 sites were laid out so that each occupant had some semblance of privacy – part of that Vermont independence thing, I guessed. Reading the park brochure, I learned that Molly was a nickname. The actual name of the lady who bore General Stark 11 children was Elizabeth.

Because of the low temperature and chilling wind we did not linger long when starting at the top of Hogsback Mountain. Trying to get warm, I ran the early downhill faster than I wanted, and I felt the pounding from this downhill jogging.

Two eye-catchers in the first couple of miles: the Vermont Dairy Goat Association and Pawsitively Perfect, catchy name for a dog grooming business, but how does the owner stay in business isolated out here in this mountain area?

At 3.5 miles a woman runner in her 20s, accompanied by her dog, yells in passing, "What a beautiful day, huh?"

"And, boy, do I appreciate it," I yelled back as she passed in the opposite direction. A once-in-a-lifetime encounter.

Speaking of such, one of the fallouts of being 80 is that when you visit places, see people, do things, you often find yourself thinking, Is this the last time for this?

By five miles I am keenly aware of a big change from the previous two days. Semis were crowding the road today, whereas there were none the previous two days – probably because they were Saturday and Sunday.

Also crowding the road were motorcycles. Yesterday at least 200 passed me, and from what I was seeing that number should be exceeded today. At Hogsback yesterday I'd talked with some motorcyclists and learned that the exodus was to races in Laconia, New Hampshire.

Every time a group of motorcyclists passed me, none waved and I was struck with the grim expressions on their faces. Maybe they were trying to reflect a macho image.

When I first saw the sign, Marlboro College, I thought it had to do with cigarettes. Later when I stopped in at the Marlboro Country Store, I learned it's actually an arts and letters college with 300 students. Imagine graduating from there and someone asks, "Where did you go to college?"

"Marlboro." Hardly an inducement to enroll there.

Just who was Colonel Williams? I was left wondering when I came upon the Colonel Williams Inn, an attractive and quaint two-story frame building, circa 1769, advertising fine dining and lodging. Very inviting.

At the Sweetbriar Country Store in Marlboro I expected to see maple syrup featured, but the advertising of Vermont cheese surprised me. I found nothing especially noteworthy about the houses and businesses, mainly restaurants, in the Marlboro area. Nothing seemed to reflect the town's proximity to a college.

Maybe I should be living in Vermont, I thought on realizing that I had not experienced any asthma problems the past four days.

Around 7.5 miles when unexpectedly I came into a flat valley, I was lulled into believing I was edging out of the hills. A heavy dose of hills a mile later dispelled that belief.

Not until around 10 miles did I work my way from the mountains into a relatively flat area. As usual after a spell of downhill running, the flat seemed almost uphill.

Once I reached the West Brattleboro, I was in a built-up area until the end of our 17.6-mile day. By now I had it right, Brattleboro, whereas my first inclination had been to call it "Battlesboro."

From his heavenly perch William Brattleboro, after whom the town is named, would not appreciate that. Incidentally Brattleboro got one hell of a real estate bargain, paying one farthing an acre–a farthing being one-quarter of a penny. At that price Bill Gates could afford to buy all of the USA.

Old Molly gets around, I concluded as I saw the Molly Stark Motel. Going past the nearby Vermont State Police building reminded me that in three days on the road I had not seen one trooper.

The building in West Brattleboro that caught my attention was the Jedediah Beal home, 1805, a two-story brick structure in mint condition. Otherwise there was nothing special about the homes in West Brattleboro, though some on the east end of town were huge, six bedrooms by my estimate.

About the same time I saw the sign, "Welcome to Brattleboro, incorporated 1753," I saw the Creamery Covered Bridge across Whetstone Brook. The bridge dates back to 1879 and still in use.

Elaine was parked nearby for a pit stop, so we took time out to photograph it and read about it. I learned that it is but one of 13 covered bridges in Windham County. Pray that does not inspire a Bridges of Windham County.

Knowing that Brattleboro is affectionately known as "the hub of New England," that it has 12,200 residents and that it is the most industrialized town in New England, I expected some congestion and traffic problems. This is exactly what I encountered at the junctions of Highway 9 and 91. Getting across 91 required some fancy footwork.

Once that was accomplished, I found myself in an area of luxury homes. I gasped when I first saw a four-story building made of stone, balcony around the front and another across the second story.

Once a palatial private home it is now the Houghton Memorial Home, established 1892, for residential care. Could this Houghton be related to the Houghton of Houghton-Mifflin?

This home for old folks set me off to thinking about age and aging. "Old age," Golda Meir once said, "is like a plane flying through a storm. Once you are aboard, there is nothing you can do."

What a crock! What a typical attitude of so many old people – people resigned to a rocking chair, to being sedentary, to succumbing to assisted-living, to being absorbed with their woes and aging.

There is plenty they can do to combat aging: exercise, think positive, have an agenda, exercise their sense of humor, have interests and ad infinitum. True, if we are lucky, we can't help getting older, but we need to recognize the difference between age (biological, chronological) and aging (a surrendering of abilities and attitudes through inactivity, physical and mental).

"I am 80 years old," said movie star Kirk Douglas. "I can't believe it... It is hard for me to realize that is reality, that I am not playing the part of an old man."

In many ways I have the same delightful problem. I don't know what is par for age 80 – who does? – but I don't think I act, feel, think, move about as 80, albeit I've slowed down in a number of ways. My enjoyment of the riches of life, my appreciation of life itself is probably fuller now than ever, something the years have increased rather than diminished.

So Kirk Douglas can't believe he's 80. When I look in a mirror, when I see myself in a video or on TV, I can't believe that's me.

That's a wrinkled, grisly, balding old man, not me. I am expecting to see the vibrant, young-at-heart person I have in my mind's eye.

It must be extremely difficult, almost depressing, for a once strikingly handsome young man as Douglas was, to look in a mirror and see an old man. Of life's many problems, that's not one I face.

To me it's more of a question of how you are old rather than of how old (the biological thing) you are. Do you wear those years with dignity or dejection? Are you alive to the wonders of life?

Too many people are aged before they ever get old. As Ben Franklin said, "Many men die at 25 and they aren't buried until they're 75."

"There is no cure for life or death," said George Santayana, "except to enjoy the interval." Too many people grow old before their years because they never find a way to enjoy the interval.

In all truth not only is it difficult for me to grasp that I am 80, but I am also immensely pleased and extremely surprised with my continued existence. But for only as long as I continue mentally alert and physically active.

As I understand it, the gerontologists ascribe old age primarily to genes. Not so in my case, I believe, for I've lived eight years beyond the genes my parents gave me.

I'm inclined to believe that what longevity I enjoy is the result of a lifetime of exercising. That's the primary factor, especially the running I've done the past 33 years. I have the idea, weird or unscientific as it might be, that the single best way to expand my life span is to exercise every day.

Whoops, maybe I should not have said that because it might lead some people to thinking that I run for longevity. Wrong. I run because I enjoy it, because it adds zest to my life in many ways.

How each person grows old is very much an individual matter, and the variance between two people of the same age can be mind boggling. That so, why does the media invariably treat aging collectively? Why does it stereotype all older people as one and the same?

One frightening aspect of aging is the rapidity with which days come and go. Sort of the feeling that you're on a roller coaster on the downhill ride and the acceleration keeps increasing as you head down toward the finish of your ride through life. Speaking of finishing, so ends my aging oration.

For a town of its size (12,200, remember) Brattleboro seemed to have an abundance of dentists and attorneys, judging from all the offices I passed on my way toward the downtown section. Since we had toured the town on the day prior to driving to Bennington and starting our west-east run, I expected no surprises as I headed for the New Hampshire border. This time, though, as apart from the first, I was better informed about the town as a result of some reading.

I knew it had no water problems by virtue of being located where the West and Connecticut rivers meet. I'd read that for a town of its size, it provides a remarkable diversity of cultural richness (art galleries, museums, theater, music), and that Rudyard Kipling built a home for his bride at nearby Dummerton and did some of his writing there. I was even well enough informed to look around (vainly) for Harris Hill ski jump, one of the few Olympic-sized 70-meter ski jumps in the USA.

And I knew the town's history dated back to 1724 with the erection of Fort Dummer, built on the present town site. The history of the fort was so well documented that there was an account of the military rations: one pound of bread and half a pint of peas or beans each day; two pounds of pork for three days, and a gallon of molasses for 42 days. Rations were augmented by fish and game as available. Nonetheless, were the rations similar in the Marine Corps, I would have considered deserting!

Having been there before, I was not surprised to see downtown Brattleboro jammed into both sides of a narrow street. The building that stood out most, at least for me, was the municipal building – three stories, brick, perched on top of a hill.

The downtown streets were overwhelmed with traffic, and the sidewalks were awash with pedestrians. Despite my antiquity, and my colorful attire of yellow T-shirt and red shorts, no one took any notice of me.

I had the feeling I could have been armed with a .45 Colt and no one would have blinked an eye. Vermont individual independence!

A half-mile from the municipal building on Highway 9 and going east I looked to my right and saw a small mountain range extending to the town's edge. So much for Brattleboro being flat.

When I passed the Fairfield Shopping Plaza, the activity thereabouts was buzzing with the same intensity I'd seen downtown. This left the impression that the economy of Brattleboro is quite healthy.

Just prior to reaching the New Hampshire boundary, I had to execute a scary maneuver when I worked my way under a subway at a curve in the road. On both sides of the road the subway cement wall came to the very edge of the road, leaving not an inch of running space except for the road itself.

I had to invade the car lane to negotiate the subway. Facing traffic, I could not see into the car lane because of the curve and the cement subway wall.

My only alternative was to cross the road and go with traffic. Not too easy a task since I had to evade 55-MPH traffic to get across. Once there I had to wait for a break in the traffic, and when it came I dashed the 100 yards under the subway and to a safe spot roadside.

Collecting myself, I saw before me the bridge over the Connecticut River that lead to the New Hampshire boundary, our finish point. Halfway across the bridge I caught sight of Elaine in the parking lot of the Riverside Motel and Restaurant.

She was waving a piece of food. Anything to get me to pick up the pace, I thought.

Describing Vermont, poet John Darling wrote:

Up where the north wind blows just a little keener,
Up where the grasses grow just a little greener,
Up where the mountain peaks rise a little higher,
Up where the human kind draws just a little nigher,
That's where Vermont comes in.

Been there, seen that, I can say, aye, and verily so! Next stop: New Hampshire

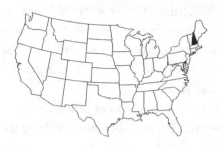

Chapter 17

New Hampshire

A Piece of Cake Compared to Vermont

Dates: *June 18th and 19th, 1997*
Miles: *33.8*
Route: *Start on Highway 2, Maine/New Hampshire border, and follow it west to Lancaster and Connecticut River, New Hampshire/ Vermont border.*

DAY ONE. In just one glance at a map of New Hampshire I saw that the shortest stretch across the state was an east-west route across the northern neck of the state. A second glance told me that Highway 2 appeared to be the best road to run in that area.

The next move was to contact a runner for his evaluation of this route. I was lucky to locate Dick Perkins, a resident of Concord, New Hampshire, who told me he's run most of the roads in the state. Dick reported, "Highway 2 is the shortest route across the state. It has paved shoulders most of the way.

"Traffic flow can be heavy in the summer but not a problem. There is only one major hill, this just to the west of Gorham. There is no big city along the route, just the small towns of Gorham and Lancaster."

Dick's report made the decision easy: Highway 2, east to west, was the New Hampshire route. By my rough calculation the border-to-border distance was close to 36 miles, which almost automatically decreed two days of 18 miles each across the state, Maine border to Vermont border.

Yesterday after we had located an RV park 4.5 miles from the

Maine border, our starting point, I got the bright idea that perhaps I could hitchhike to the border, then run back the 4.5 miles to the RV park and be that far ahead the next day (today) when we actually started. Alas, that did not come to pass because I failed to get a ride to the start. I stood in front of the RV park 45 minutes trying to hitch to the border.

More than 50 drivers passed me, but none offered me a ride. So I gave up the idea of getting a head start.

Standing roadside and failing to get a ride, I remembered back to my college days at University of California, Berkeley, and hitchhiking the 90 miles home every couple of weeks and never failing to get a ride. Times change, or is it that the moods of people change with the times?

In the starting area this morning the word that came to mind was comfort. I was in the fabulous running setting of a nine-foot breakdown lane with newly surfaced blacktop, about as good as it gets on the road.

I hadn't gone very far when I was made aware that we were relatively close to Canada, as I saw a sign posted in both English and French. The word "Avis" was the heading on the sign, and just as I was thinking, What's Avis car rental doing out here?, my high school French came to my rescue. I realized that the word means "notice," leaving me feeling sort of foolish for having the Avis car rental thought.

Another sign, this one near two ponds, caught my attention: "Moose Crossing." Going past the ponds, I was relieved not to see a moose on the loose.

However, when I came to the Shelburne town waste disposal area and realized the fascination bears have for garbage dumps, my eyeballs went on bear patrol since I was aware that bears are known to be about in this region.

Got some evidence that New Hampshire is heavy into the lumber industry when, just a few yards off the highway, I saw considerable action around a huge chipping enterprise. Enough logs were stacked up to fill three or four football fields. Exhibit B of lumber playing a big role in the state's economy was that in every direction I looked all I saw was small mountains, heavily forested– even more so than Vermont.

Around 1.5 miles I was actually thankful that what had been a mist when we started had transcended into rain. I had been buzzed by squadrons of mosquitoes, but now the rain grounded them.

About all I saw going through the village of Shelburne were eight homes, a cemetery and a gas station. A sign pointed to the village center off to the north. Looking in that direction, I could see a church steeple, an elementary school, a few residences, golf course and a city park.

In the Shelburne area I passed a quarter-mile long , 60 or more feet high bluff of granite that told me this is why New Hampshire is called the "Granite State."

Just how many times have I come upon the Appalachian Trail this summer, I asked myself as I went by a parking area for hikers using the trail. Looking at the mountains on both sides of the road, being in the fog, heavy forestation all about, was remindful to me of being in the Humboldt Redwoods area in northern California.

Around 4.5 miles my honeymoon with the comfort of a breakdown lane and newly surfaced blacktop lane ended, and I found myself confined to a narrow shoulder.

No reason, though, to break out the boo-hoo handkerchiefs. After all, the running conditions were still good compared to the vicissitudes of Vermont with its narrow road, mountains, sightless curves and heavy traffic.

On the bridge over the Rattle (not for rattlesnakes, I hoped) River I paused a couple of minutes to absorb the view 100 yards on each side of the bridge. A touch of fascination as I watched the clear, fast flowing water cascading over huge boulders.

I can understand the guy who danced with wolves because here I was talking to a huge stone home build in 1854. Been sitting here 114 years, baby, and I'd bet that you've never seen an 80-year old runner in his BVD's pass by and, what's more, comment on what a charming lady you are! Oh, the stories you could tell!

For her second pit stop Elaine was parked near the Town and Country Motor Inn, an extravagant resort spread over 300 yards. Across the street was the golf course of the Androscoggin Valley Country Club.

Elaine decided to walk the dogs on a path adjacent to the golf course. As she was doing so, a golfer driving a golf cart sped up to her, braked and said, "Oh geez, I thought I was going to see a moose!" Yeah, we gotta put those dogs on a diet!

One of the best treats for me in the Gorham area was the views of the Presidential Mountains. There are a number of them, and I list them alphabetically to keep this devoid of politics: Adams, Eisenhower, Franklin Jackson, Jefferson, Madison, Monroe, Pierce and Washington (at 6288 feet, the highest point in New Hampshire).

Franklin being included confused me. Did it represent Franklin Roosevelt or Ben Franklin? If old Ben, why was he elevated to presidential status?

Another treat in Gorham was indulging in a Boston cream donut that Elaine rescued from Dunkin Donuts. After that fix I was primed for the day!

When I went past one inn today and saw a sign about a 50th wedding anniversary, my thoughts went to Richard and Margaret Kegley, who celebrated their 50th wedding anniversary by running the Portland Marathon together. Got me to wondering if they are the only couple to ever celebrate a 50th wedding anniversary by running a 26.2-mile race. I'd cast a "yes" vote on that.

Gorham was loaded with motels, restaurants and shops. A bit of overkill here, I thought, as I saw about 30 percent of the businesses displaying moose decorations and signs of various designs. Seeing houses and businesses interspersed, I got the impression that zoning is loose.

Best as I could detect, only two fast food franchises–Pizza Hut and the ever-present McDonald's – have invaded Gorham. Since the town has only 3000 residents, these invaders bespeak of heavy tourism.

To me the most unusual sight in town was the backyard of a home completely filled with graves, some having been there for 150 years. Across the street was the city cemetery. Pretty hard to pass by here, the corner of Main and Norman Streets, without giving a thought to death.

Wonder how close they get to Mt. Washington, was my thought as I passed an airport where biplane rides were offered to adventurous tourists? Some place I'd read that Mt. Washington is one of the windiest places in the world, which considerably reduced the appeal of buzzing around the mountain in a biplane.

Was glad to be peeled down to shorts and a T-shirt when, west of Gorham, I came upon the hill Dick Perkins had described. By my reckoning it was about one mile long and of an eight-percent gradient.

Enough to roust my dormant asthma from its slumber.

As I started up the hill, I caught sign of another "Moose Crossing" sign. I also saw a cement wall built to deter the moose from crossing.

The wall sort of conveyed the idea that the moose were out and about. Yeah, probably so, but so far the only wildlife I've seen today was a jack rabbit scampering across the road.

On top of the hill a roadside sign reading, "Randolph. Population 371." All I saw roadside was a church. When I asked about Randolph, I learned that it is a summer-cottage colony at the northern edge of the Presidential Range.

Speaking of learning things, when I paid our RV lodging bill last night, the manager explained, "We have an eight-percent tax on lodging and meals. But we have no state income tax, no sales or use tax and no automobile sales tax."

So, a tax on lodging and meals – sort of a slick way, I concluded, to shift the tax burden from the residents to the tourists.

Near the end of our 18.8-mile day I was exalting over the good feeling of experiencing strength coming into my running. The reason was simple: By now I have been on the road long enough this year to begin to feel the buildup.

Several times today I found myself thinking back on an article I'd read last night, a report that there are 3.5 million millionaires in our country. Asking myself how many of these I know, I had to strain myself to come up with 10, two of whom are now dead.

The most interesting one was a friend of my mother's who frequented the resort where she worked. He owned a wrecking company in a metropolitan area.

What was unusual about him was that he could neither read nor write. But he had a gift for looking at a building, analyzing it and accurately estimating what it would cost to demolish it.

Through running I've met at least three millionaires, and with a couple of them I've had humorous experiences. The first was with a business man who was involved in staging a race, a community service on his part.

He called me long distance to tell me about the race, to ask some questions about race management and to persuade me to enter the race. The long-distance call had gone on quite a while and – not knowing he was a millionaire and worried about his mounting phone bill – I said, "This call is costing you plenty. Maybe I should write the answers to some of the information you want."

"No need to be concerned," he replied. "The race can handle it."

The other experience, again through running, with a millionaire who happened to be a runner. After we'd finished a 20-mile training run together, he said, "Let's go to lunch."

"Good idea," I said. I understood we'd go Dutch treat, and I expected a good restaurant as a reward for our 20-mile workout. "Where do you want to go?" I asked.

"How about Dairy Queen?" he said.

The guy's gotta be kidding, I told myself. He wasn't, and I decided that if going the Dairy Queen route is the price to become a millionaire, my reaction, in Samuel Goldwyn's immortal words, was, "Include me out."

From a distance I've observed a former student of mine who has become a millionaire. My observation has been that as his fortune grew, his love of money kept growing.

He's now a slave to money. His central focus in life is to add to his fortune, to watch his money grow.

John Lennon once said something about too many people passing through life without living. Despite his big bucks, this guy is in that category.

Then I thought of another millionaire I know who's a recluse. She goes out only to buy groceries or to shop in a department store.

Travel, theater, movies, concerts or other cultural events are not on her agenda. Fact is, she doesn't even attend church. Seems like an awful waste of a life – and money.

For sure, Arnold Schwarzenegger, with whom I've talked three or four times (he chairs the California Governor's Council on Physical Fitness and Sports to which I am a consultant), is a millionaire. When Arnold learned that I was about to attempt to run across the country, he sent a huge floral piece with a note reading, "Good luck on your massive trek." Arnold's act reflects one of the reasons I'd like to be a millionaire – to use the money to bring pleasure into the lives of people.

"Money's like an arm or a leg, use it or lose it," Henry Ford told us. If I had not seen examples, I'd find it difficult to believe some millionaires don't use it.

Now that's where I'd be normal; I'd have no trouble there, and I'd spend much of it lighting up the lives of others. But no matter how rich I was, I'd be a common man, no fancy airs–yes, even as a humble man – as evidenced by the fact that I'd be seen frequenting Round Table Pizza, Dunkin Donuts, In/Out Burgers and Baskin Robbins.

In no way would my humility extend to the Golden Arches.

DAY TWO. Always a good feeling to wake up and know that if the day goes well Elaine and I will succeed in crossing another state. Even though the distance across a state is short, the feeling of achievement is always there. Obviously, though, not to the same degree as longer states, such as Kansas at 499 miles.

When I was paying the RV park manager last night, I told him about how much I enjoyed the views of the Presidential Range. "Actually," he said, "they're not the most popular mountains in the state. Monadnock down the south part of the state is the second most popular mountain in the world for climbing, right behind Mount Fuji."

"How high is it?" I asked.

"Oh, around 3,200 feet," he replied.

Didn't seem very high to me, and I was left wondering what the attraction was but I didn't ask. Maybe just because it was an easy climb.

Our talking about mountains brought to mind a comparison Robert Frost made between those in Vermont and New Hampshire. Something to the effect that the Vermont mountains are straight and the New Hampshire mountains are curled up in a coil. That comparison was about all I could recall from his Pulitzer Prize-winning poem "New Hampshire" except for the fact that it covered about 15 pages and that, for me, it did not have the appeal of some of his other poems.

This was another one of those days when we got a late start. Delaying us were the 15-mile drive to the start, stopping at the post office in Gorham, photographing in Gorham (my favorite: a wooden moose carved to scale) and ducking into Dunkin Donuts to get Elaine a chocolate donut. The conservative type, I settled for glazed.

Starting, I expected to get drenched. Rain was on the scene constantly for the past 15 hours, and I started in a light rain. Mercifully it ceased after I'd gone five miles. The day remained overcast but considerably kinder than I had anticipated.

This was one of those days when there was always a structure of some sort in sight. The route was saturated with motels, hotels, restaurants and gift shops. So much so that it was hard to believe that 80 percent of the state still remains forested.

However, New Hampshire ran a distant second to Vermont with vendors of local crafts and products.

One of the most unusual sights of the day, and this within my first three miles, was a stone building about 40 feet high. It had several floors, each about the size of one large room and each with windows.

There was a front-door entrance and an observation tower. A footpath lead to the entrance. There was no evidence of a driveway or any vehicle accommodation. The feeling I had was that exploring here would be more interesting than a trip to Disneyland.

Two attractions along the way caught me by surprise, probably because they seemed out of character for New Hampshire. Well, that's wrong: out of character for forested New Hampshire but very hep for touristy New Hampshire.

Both were in the area east of Jefferson, and I'd guess about midway between Gorham and Lancaster. The first one I saw was Six Gun City, and that's just what it was: a frontier city.

But not entirely: It was embellished with a miniature golf course, waterslides (from a quarter-mile away I could hear the riders screaming) and other money-makers.

The second attraction was Santa's Village. All the Christmas hoopla was there, plus a monorail and a roller coaster (where the riders out-screamed those at Six Gun City).

Going past, I caught sight of a young couple escorting 20 preschool children. Seated in the parking lot beside their bus, they were devouring their bag lunches. My thought: Disneyland would not let you do that.

Another sight that drew my attention, this at six miles when I came to Starr King Cemetery on top of a hill and there I saw a grave site built into the side of a hill. Entrance was through a wooden door which appeared to be unlocked (irrelevant, though, because I had not the slightest desire to enter). As I moved on, I wondered if this would meet code specifications in a metropolitan city.

Elaine was envious this morning when I saw a moose that she had missed. When I first saw it in a pond, I thought it was too big to be a moose, then it moved and it was easily detectable as a moose.

As it moved, I saw a calf trailing it. I had expected more of a brown color but what I saw was sort of a henna.

When I came into the motorhome for the nine-mile pit stop, Elaine asked, "What do you want?". Let's spice up the day, I told myself, and not give her a routine answer and said instead, "Oh, some tapioca pudding with a sprinkle of bananas and canned cherries on top, with a glazed donut on the side, and a Pepsi to drink."

"So you're delusioning again," she said. "In that case, what you want is what I give you." So much for spice.

Two towns were on today's route, Jefferson and Lancaster. Jefferson consisted of two inns, two general stores, 20 or so residences, a post office, an elementary school and a town square with a World War II memorial. On the west end of town was a small hospital; for sure, no open-heart surgery here.

The two most elaborate structures were the three story Manor Motel and the Hillside Inn. The nearby Jefferson History Society Museum, housed in an old church building, posted a sign, "Open Sundays only." Talk about bad luck because I was all in a dither about touring it.

The most notable feature of Lancaster was all the charming homes, many of them old and wearing the years with elegance. One, I was told, went back to 1780.

Lancaster, settled in 1764, is proud of being the first town in Northern New Hampshire. The setting is picturesque, in a valley surrounded by mountains at the confluence of the Connecticut and Israel Rivers. Despite that vintage the town has a population of only 3500.

For such a small town it seemed to have a number of parks. At Soldier's Park I paused to read a memorial to the dead of all wars in which Lancaster residents were killed.

At Mechanic Street when I looked to my right, I saw one of the state's many covered bridges, but I was not about to make a six block round-trip out of my way for a closer look. To paraphrase a native son, one Robert Frost. "miles to go before I finish."

In the middle of town while going past a small hill, I saw that it was home to what I'd call a boot hill cemetery. Sort of a reminder of how old the town is, and located so that 90 percent of tourists driving by would miss it.

Passing a real estate office, I paused to look at pictures of homes for sale and to study prices. They seemed more reasonable than California homes.

Kind of amusing to me that, amid all the antiquity and history, I came across four pizza joints within four blocks. On second thought I might be defaming them by calling them joints because three days ago on the drive eastward we stopped in one, Scorpio's. I drooled when saying the name again because the pizza was one of the very best I've ever tasted.

Very refreshing to wander through Lancaster on the sidewalks and not have to worry about the crown of the road or oncoming vehicles embracing me.

I had two running problems today. The first was the many loggers on the road, driving with a frenzy and leading me to suspect they were paid by the load. As they sped towards me, I scampered to safety.

My second problem was a badly bruised heel. I padded it with moleskin, then wrapped elastoplast tape over the moleskin. I tried to offset the injury by landing on the ball of my foot instead of the heel and also by trying to pretend I had a cortisone shot for it. But every time my foot struck, I felt like yelling, "Yikes!"

I also knew that the miles would stack up faster and easier, and the pain would be less, if I could do some disassociating - get my mind off running and sort of space out with other thoughts. But I had a problem trying to get my mind off running because every time my bruised left heel hit the ground, I winced in pain.

The main focus of my disassociating was on weakness or handicap, or whatever, of mine: music: I have no sense of what I call "rhythm" and what my friend and college roommate Bill Glackin, a highly respected arts critic for the Sacramento Bee, calls "timing."

When I listen to a band - no matter how good, Basie, Ellington, Goodman - I can't pick up the beat. This doesn't keep me from enjoying the music, but it has been a big handicap in life in a couple of ways.

First, women: Without timing, I am a lousy dancer, something that was always a handicap in my dating days.

Even today I regret the deficiency because I know Elaine likes to dance.

Desperate on that score, I've often thought of asking her to do the leading and I'd learn to follow, for which timing would be helpful but not necessary if I've got it right. But I have yet to ask or try this.

Second, the Marine Corps: Parades, to me, are one step short of combat. Try as I might, I could never distinguish the beat of the band.

I simply followed the others, which meant that I usually had my eyes on the ground (oops, deck) instead of straight ahead – a Marine Corps sin unto itself. But there came a time in my Marine Corps career when I could no longer follow others.

As a battalion commander I stood in front of 1200 troops. I was lined up directly behind the band, and when it struck up my duty was to yell, "Forward!"

That I could do, no sense of timing required. But the next step I could not do even if my life depended on it.

That step called for me to yell, precisely at the 16th count of the music, "March!" That command required timing, and it was important because the battalion stepped off on that count. I worked my way around that by having my adjutant, directly behind me, yell the command.

As the band stepped off, I had no problem. Just follow their steps.

My problem descended when the band turned out (made a sudden left turn when I continued straight) just before the reviewing stand. Suddenly I was naked, no one in front of me, the band playing – all blah, blah to me.

I was supposed to maintain the cadence. And compounding the problem, we were about to pass the reviewing stand and I had to give a command, "Eyes Right!" to my staff directly behind me – at which time they and I, while continuing to move straight head, must execute a maneuver that called for us to point our swords 90 degrees to the right of our bodies while looking at the reviewing stand.

All of which triggered a degree of panic in me: thoughts such as try to maintain cadence, don't drop the sword (and many have), don't swerve to the right, focus on continuing straight (hey, pick a landmark dead ahead!). Those seconds as I passed the review stand marched by in Indian file.

Understandably, I envy people born with the gift of timing, something most probably don't recognize as a gift, and I often wonder what caused me to be without it.

The disassociating must have worked well because when I rounded a turn on the west edge of Lancaster, I saw the green steel beams of the bridge over the Connecticut River. My reaction was, Here so soon?

Once across the bridge and the river I was in Vermont. Going across the bridge I found myself marveling over the fact that as far back as 1764 the King of England had fixed the Connecticut River as the boundary between New Hampshire and Vermont.

Waiting for me, Elaine was parked in front of an old barn that had been converted to an antiques and collectibles store. I was fascinated with a body-armor suit, the type worn by King Arthur's knights, that was reasonably priced.

"Don't even think about it," Elaine said, squashing my chance to be knighted.

Our running day over, I coaxed Elaine into going back to Scorpio's so that I could confirm the pizza there was as good as I remembered. It was.

We spent the night in Lancaster on the shores of the Connecticut River, which by now was becoming an old friend.

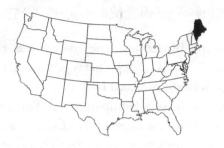

Chapter 18

Maine

Another Finish in the Atlantic

Date: *June 21st, 1997*
Miles: *19.1*
Route: *Start on Highway 9, New Hampshire/Maine border, and follow 9 east to Wells Beach, Atlantic Ocean, east border of Maine..*

Catalog shopping through L.L. Bean was about as close as I got to Maine before planning to run across the state. My original plan called for a west-east run on Highway 25, finishing at Portland – the state's biggest city, albeit having a population of only 65,000.

This plan was reinforced when George Towle, a coach at the University of Southern Maine, (which happens to be along the Highway 25 route) told me this was a feasible road for running.

But that plan got torpedoed when we happened to check out Highway 9, another west-east route across the state, on our way north to Highway 25. Scouting 9, we found that it was shorter than 25, had a runnable shoulder practically all the way and the traffic flow (except in the beach area) was no problem. Jilting Highway 25 for 9 was an easy decision, though we did regret this meant we would not get a look at Portland.

The New Hampshire/Maine boundary, our starting point, was distinctly marked on a bridge over the Salmon Falls River. The town of Berwick appeared to be located on both sides of the river, but the actual location was Maine. However, with the naked eye there was no way of knowing it did not extend into New Hampshire.

I actually started about 60 yards inside of New Hampshire, to the west of the bridge, simply because that was the closest spot to the border that Elaine could find to park the motorhome and unload me. As I got underway, I knew that the battle plan called for me to cover a spit over 19 miles and finish Maine in one day; I knew that this was one of the kindest routes this year (no big hills, no sightless curves, moderate traffic, runnable shoulder practically all the way), and I was aware that if all went well the climax of the day would be a seafood dinner at Wells Beach – lobster for Elaine, crab cakes for me. Well, at least I hoped that – and not some disaster – would be the climax.

What a whale of a difference between today when I headed for the Atlantic and when, seven years ago, I left the Pacific Ocean in California and headed for the Atlantic. Today I had only 19 miles to go and I'd be crossing my 45th state. Leaving California, I had 3192 miles to go and I was crossing my first state.

The 1990 run was my apprenticeship. Now I am a journeyman.

One of the first places I passed today was the Pine Tanning Factory. The sign over the gate read, "Through these gates pass the best leather makers in the world." Okay, note here, oh seasoned traveler, that leather is part of the Maine economy.

This is only the second morning this year when the weather has permitted me to start in T-shirt and shorts. But on many of the mornings when I started bundled, a young stud would be comfortable in T-shirt and shorts. Okay, note here, oh youthful ones, that one of the ravages of old age is an intolerance for the cold.

As I went past the Berwick Middle School, I observed its resemblance to other middle schools I'd seen in New England: sturdily built, three stories, brick. This one dated back to 1927. My thought: Would it pass as a safe building under the California legal requirements for earthquake proof buildings?

Before we left home this summer, a friend of Elaine's had forewarned us, "Watch out for the rattlesnakes in Maine. They're huge and plentiful."

I thought about him as I went past a dead snake at 1.5 miles. I examined the snake, saw that he had a viper head, gray circles around his body, a brownish-copper coloring and some black spots between the circles. His tail was so badly smashed by a car that I could not make out whether or not he had rattles.

Working my way up a hill while still in the built-up area, I stopped

to photograph one of the many big homes along the way. Why, I
wondered, so many big homes in New England? Big by my standard
was five or six bedrooms.

Once out of the built-up area and moseying along, I settled into a
comfortable pace, and the environment also being comfortable I
became a spectator of the passing scene:

- The name of one of the local newspapers, *Foster's Daily
  Democrat*, seemed a bit oddball to me. I had yet to read this
  paper. I learned its name from seeing it on paper receptacles in
  front of each home.
- Caught sight of a backyard with a clothesline full of laundry
  and realized this was becoming a familiar sight in New
  England. Why so many washings hanging in the breeze? Was
  this New England frugality? Maybe the people can't afford a
  dryer? Could skyrocket prices for utilities be the reason? Or do
  the folks simply prefer the fresh smell of clothes dried by the
  sun and the wind? Some profound considerations here. Calls
  for a Ph.D. study in sociology.
- Seeing gobs of pine trees, I could easily understand why Maine
  is called the "Pine State." They are so closely bunched that it is
  more dark than light beneath them.
- Ah, we do have a touch of culture in these parts as evidenced
  by a sign advertising that "Carousel" will be opening at the
  Hackmatack Playhouse June 24th.
- Also evidence of agriculture along the way as I passed a couple
  of hay fields. Caught off guard on that one because I had
  expected to see potatoes (only Idaho and Washington produce
  more spuds than Maine) or blueberries (here Maine leads the
  nation in production).
- A sign, "38 acres, $29,900." Nice-looking area, pine trees and
  woodsy. Can that be the total price?
- A black mark for Maine: This highway has more litter than any
  road I saw in Vermont, New Hampshire or Connecticut.
- Another sign, "Deer Cutting." At one time I knew what that
  meant, but as I went past it I couldn't even guess at its meaning.
- A Pratt Whitney engine plant stirred up memories of scouting
  missions in torpedo bombers that were powered by Pratt
  Whitneys.

- Seemed that during the last eight miles today there was a garage sale about every mile. Could this be a case of the locals enticing cash from the tourists?
- Highway 9 was similar to many other roads recently traveled – apparently no zoning judging from the fact that homes and businesses were interspersed.

Somewhat surprised not to see any deer in the wooded areas. Didn't expect, though, to see any moose since we'd seen no moose crossing signs when scouting this route.

On the other hand, I wasn't sure the moose were aware they were not expected to cross this road. From what I'd read, moose are plentiful in Maine but they inhabit the northern part of the state.

One interesting fact that I learned about them is that their six-foot antlers can weigh up to 90 pounds. Could be that a heavy dose of Tylenol might help them get through a day.

The Maine license plates have "Vacationland" across the bottom of them. So be it, but anyone heading for these parts better be able to deal with humidity. On this particular day I felt as if I were in a sauna, he said with profuse apologies to the Maine Chamber of Commerce.

Even though I had my bruised left heel padded with moleskin and wrapped with elastoplast tape, it troubled me – reminding me uncomfortably so with each strike of my left foot that it was not disposed to running today. Other than the irksome heel I had no physical problems, the road was accommodating enough, and most of the Maine drivers moved over when they saw me.

If I had any problem today, it was that entertainment was hard to come by. There was no spectacular scenery, no striking sights and no conversations with any of the citizenry. In fact, when seven bicyclists went past, I waved and said "Hi," but they remained as silent as that noted Maine resident, Calvin Coolidge.

With little to see and with safe running conditions, I resorted to ruminating. First came some thoughts about our society, then some thoughts about the most formative years of my life.

About our society I juggled an assortment of thoughts, all on the downbeat side and all entertaining me but briefly:

- That people who burn the flag should be deported.
- That people who refuse to pledge allegiance to the flag should lose their citizenship. Yes, both those reactions are, by most

standards, extreme; by ACLU standards, radical I'm sure. Some-where, though, if a country, if a government is to survive, a line has to be drawn. My line is drawn out of reverence for American war dead.

• That discipline and courtesy are direly needed throughout our society.

• That despite all the yakking and studies about improving education, little or no recognition is given to the fundamental need or problem of education – to wit, a learning environment must exist in the classroom.

Somber as all that thinking was, it was fleeting. What I dwelled on went back to and remained focused on were my first three years of high school, 1932 – 1934, back 65 years, hard as that is to believe.

These were the most formative years of my life, though I did not realize it at the time. Years when I was closest to God, years when I learned how to study, years when I began to appreciate learning and knowledge, and years when my character began to take shape.

Closest to God because I was in a religious setting. I was one of 50 boys studying to be a member of the religious order of the Christian Brothers. I thought I had what is called a "vocation." Considering that the Brothers had taken care of me all the time I was progressing through grades two to eight – all of which I spent 24 hours a day boarding at one of their schools – and considering they were my heroes, it would seem to be quite understandable that I wanted to be one of them.

The focus of our daily lives was on things spiritual–mass and communion at six A.M., listening at each of our three meals to readings from the lives of the saints (every boy took a turn at reading), an hour of catechism daily, benediction and prayers in the evening. Augmenting this spiritual focus was our being isolated eight miles from the nearest town – no worldly distractions.

We were cut off from the world – no radio, no newspapers, no magazines; the only time we left our sanctuary was for a two-week visit home during the summer. But we were not allowed home for Christmas, Thanksgiving, or Easter.

Looking back, I realized that the key to my learning to study, to growing to appreciate learning was the guidance of Brother Pius. His secular name was, so I found out years later and only by reading it on a tombstone, was Paul Figueroa. Somehow he transmitted his enthusiasm for learning to me, always encouraging, never failing to recognize achievement and always seeking excellence.

And there was plenty to learn. No frills in the curriculum, just solid subjects – the daily schedule consisting of French, Latin, math, history, science and English (literature and composition). I didn't recognize it at the time but I do now that learning was accelerated by the competition among us and by the fact that we had little else to do.

Sort of smiled when I remembered one of the rituals. It was called "ads," and it happened every Friday night.

All 50 boys were seated in the study hall and Brother Patrick, the prefect, was at a desk in the front of the room. He would call a boy's name, which was his cue to stand.

Whereupon hunting season began because every one of the other 49 boys could tell him what he was doing wrong. The procedure was to say, "It seems to me my very dear [boy's name] that..."

As examples, "It seems to me my very dear Paul that you can't control your temper." Or, "It seems to me my very dear James that you should not chew your food with your mouth open."

The boy stood until Brother Patrick told him to be seated and in some cases, the "my very dears" flying, the standing time was long. In the course of the evening every boy stood and heard himself assailed.

The exercise was a big step in character development. Proof that the system worked was that by the time a boy reached his junior year he heard few, if any, "my very dears," whereas in his freshman year he was deluged with them. Boy, was I!

Sixty-five years, yet I have never forgotten nor will I ever forget the day the Jesuit priest in charge of the choir had each of the 50 boys individually sing the scales. When my turn came, he could not believe what he was hearing.

At first he accused me of being disruptive, of trying to ham up the scales and being clownish. Then when he realized I could not carry a tune if my life depended on it, he dismissed me as hopeless.

As a result, when the other 49 boys practiced for choir, I was told to go to the gym and practice basketball. No wonder I made the varsity as a sophomore!

Even to this day I'm not sure why I left that environment at the end of my junior year. The generic reason was that I no longer felt I had a "vocation". One thing I do know for sure is that after three years in that setting, when I returned to a regular high school for my senior year, girls were strange specimens!

Over those three years there was much family loneliness, some sacrifices and some deprivations. But as I view these years in the mirror of life, and I am grateful for them. They and Brother Pius fashioned my life.

Very few young people leave a family setting to grow and develop in the type of setting I lived in for three years. They, not I, are the average. But they, too, go through formative years during which, so I'd surmise, an array of forces mold or warp them.

Oh hell, that was too complex to think about right now. Besides, it was time to get back to the business of running.

Nearing the end of my 19.1-mile day, I again had a guilty feeling about going such a short distance and calling it across a "state." Yet technically it was, from the state's western boundary at New Hampshire to its eastern boundary at the Atlantic.

Look at it this way, I told myself, even with the short distances across some states, I will have logged more than 7600 miles across 50 states. That's a heap of miles. Really, I told myself in self-justification, no need to apologize for that.

Rounding a corner, I saw a landmark ahead, I-95, and it told me I was closing in on the ocean. Once I went under the I-95 overpass and turned south on Highway 1, I was in touristland – the entire area was wall-to-wall motels, restaurants, stores, shopping centers and bumper-to-bumper traffic.

People were everywhere, almost all of them tourists – or so I judged from their garb. All the motels and inns in this town, Wells, posted "No Vacancy" signs. It was rare to see a person on the street who was not eating some sort of snack (mainly ice cream cones) or not sipping on some soft drink.

The only building along the way that I took note of was the Wells Auto Museum. In fact, I stopped to take a picture of the historic tractor in front of it because my grandson, Scott Granlund, is fascinated with tractors and I thought he'd enjoy seeing this one.

Our destination was Wells Beach and the Atlantic Ocean. After going about a mile south along Highway 1, I came to One Mile Road, the only road leading to Wells Beach.

I really didn't enjoy that last mile for a number of reasons: mainly because the fast-flowing traffic along the narrow road posed a threat, and because the route itself, a half-mile of the built-up road being through a marsh area, was not attractive.

I also had some concern about Elaine and her problems with a motorhome in a heavily congested area with poor roadways. Her driving the motorhome in that area was akin to someone trying to do a waltz among dancers propelling themselves around to the beat of heavy-metal music.

When I reached the beach area, I saw Elaine standing there, waving to me. "I told the parking-lot attendant what I was doing," she explained, "and he was merciful and said I could park without paying the $7 until you arrived. But he said to make it quick."

And make it quick, we did. We simply took a couple of photos at the ocean's edge, then escaped the crowded Wells Beach area as fast as we could.

Come evening, the climax to the day was as Elaine had hoped: a lobster dinner. I was not so lucky because the restaurant did not serve my much anticipated crab cakes. Instead I had to settle for jumbo stuffed shrimp, but I suffered nobly!

When we turned in for the night, I was feeling – and this for about the first time best as I could remember – that we were closing in our summer goal. Only New York, Michigan and Wisconsin remained to be run on this trip, and in that order.

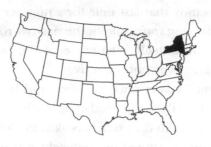

Chapter 19

New York

Back to Lake Erie Once Again

Dates: *June 25th to 26th, 1997*
Miles: *26.9*
Route: *Start at Pennsylvania/New York border on Highway 76 (Chautauqua County Road 33) and follow it north to its junction with Highway 304. Take 304 northwest until it intersects Lake Erie, New York's north border.*

DAY ONE. Contemplating running across New York, I had visions of areas crowded with cars, people and buildings. When I asked Arnold Edson, a New York resident and Marine Corps classmate, about running routes across the state, he proposed a couple of interesting routes. Both, because of extended mileage, were too ambitious for me.

Arnold also suggested, "Why not run the length of Long Island? That's about 110 miles."

That, too, sounded congested. And besides, I was looking for something shorter than 110 miles.

Studying the New York map, I saw that the shortest distance across the state was in the western part of the state, on a north-south (or south-north if you prefer) route. At first blush, the Buffalo-Niagara Falls complex looked inviting. Then remembering a visit there last year and seeing the area overrun with tourists, I backed off.

As I focused on the western part of the state, two north-south routes jumped out: Highway 62 from the Pennsylvania border to Lake Erie, via Jamestown and Fredonia; Highway 76 at the Pennsylvania border, north to Highway 394 and Chautauqua and then following 394 to Lake Erie.

I chose the Chautauqua route mainly because it was shorter. In retrospect, had I to do it over, I'd start on 62, follow it to Jamestown, then take 394 to Lake Erie. This would add distance, but it would also hold more attractions and distractions along the way.

Calculating the Pennsylvania-Chautauqua-Lake Erie route to be approximately 27 miles, I decided to split the run into two easy days.

The first thing we noted as we left I-17 and drove toward the starting area was that the AAA map and the road signs we were seeing did not agree. The AAA map showed our route as Highway 76, but the signs we saw read State Highway 33.

This was truly a day when a reconnaissance paid off because as we were driving the 76/33 route to the start, we discovered that a bridge had been washed out. The detour to our start area added about 10 miles to our route.

At the bridge site I noticed that the workmen had built a foot-bridge of planks across the stream. If they'll let me cross on that, I won't have to run those extra 10 miles, I told myself.

I explained to Jay Wilcox, foreman of the Chautauqua County Highway Department crew, what I was up to and then asked if he'd let me use the footbridge.

"No problem," he said. "Just make sure to be careful and when you get back here to cross it, make sure someone in my crew keeps an eye on you."

I thanked him profusely, and we drove the detour to reconnect with our route and to get to the start. On the way I thought of how easy it would have been for Wilcox to say "no." My experience has been that hands-on guys like him are bent to define the task and find the most expeditious way to do it (in my case, directly across the foot-bridge instead of detouring), whereas many white-collar paper shufflers would say, "We can't let you cross the footbridge. Too much liability. Company policy. I'm sorry."

I started on Highway 76/33 at the Pennsylvania/New York boundary in the Chautauqua-Allegheny region of the state. The hills were a radical departure from the stereotyped impression of New York–that being Manhattan, Statue of Liberty, United Nations Building and Broadway. This setting was light years removed from the Big Apple. One thing all our driving around the state reminded us of is that New York is a state of dramatic contrasts with the variations of the Big

Apple, the Catskills, the Adirondacks, Niagara Falls and all such.

I had expected to be on a curvy and narrow road. Instead I was pleasantly surprised to be on a mostly straight road with two lanes and a runnable shoulder. There were some hills but nothing strenuous.

In the first mile I was beginning to wonder what I had gotten myself into when I went past a place that looked like a scene out of "Deliverance." Then a short distance later I saw two pens about 30 yards off the road and filled with German Shepherds barking and running about wildly.

They were so huge that I had to look twice to confirm they were dogs and not wolves. Typical of what I was seeing in this early going, the area around the pen and the pens themselves were a mess.

All the housing in the first three miles was marginal. For sure, this was not prosperity row.

"Welcome to Panama," read the sign. The last time I saw a similar sign I was on a Princess Cruise through the Panama Canal, and it cost me considerably more than this jaunt. There I was a spectator; here I am a participant, a role much preferable.

Panama, New York, housed a midget post office, country store, garage, Junior's Restaurant and a huge Baptist church. Some of the homes in Panama looked as if they were on their deathbed.

As I passed the Needles Propane Service and saw a guy working there, I greeted him with, "Good morning. How are you doing?"

The young guy in his 30s looked at me as if to say, "Get lost, kook!"

A short while later when a farmer driving a tractor passed by, I waved to him. He acknowledged my presence in no way. I was beginning to conclude that the natives are not sociable.

Once I got beyond the Panama vicinity, the quality and neatness of the roadside homes improved dramatically and remained so upgraded for the rest of the day.

Traditional thinking would proclaim that after a few days away from running while driving to New York, I'd be strengthened and refreshed this morning. But that has rarely been my experience.. Always after a layoff I find it difficult to groove back into running. I think it's called "inertia."

Now there's a different twosome, was my thought when I saw a horse and a llama side by side. I yelled to them, "Looks like you're good neighbors."

Hearing me, they ambled to the fence. Ah, at last, some sociable natives. But I was wary of getting close. Llamas, I've been told, are prone to spit on people.

I had only one problem today. It was not with the road, which was runnable, or with the traffic, which was very light. This problem was with horse flies.

At the start area when she'd walked the dogs, Elaine returned to the motorhome where I was readying to leave and complained about horse flies. Despite that alert I neglected to spray myself with Avon bath oil, and I paid the price for this neglect as horse flies used me for a landing pad during the first three miles until I reached the motorhome for a pit stop. I guessed they were biting, but it felt more like I was being stung.

I'd like to be dramatic and report that when I came to the stream and footbridge, the crossing was perilous with water moccasins and alligators all about – both of which I evaded only by being fleet of foot. But the fact of the matter was that the only drama in the crossing was that I had to stay entirely concentrated on maintaining my balance on the plank. Once I was across the stream and on my way, the rendezvous with Elaine, who'd driven the extended detour, was accomplished in 25 minutes.

An incident at one pit stop today led me to deduce that my pit crew captain Elaine is losing some of her angelic attributes. Suddenly taken with a cramp in my left calf I stood up, yelped in pain, tried to massage it out, then turned to Elaine for tea and sympathy.

Her reply was, "Just a little bit of adversity. You can rise above it."

At the moment I wished I could e-mail Pete League and give him a message about this woman whom he dubbed a saint.

Darn thing's got the same markings as one I saw in Maine, was my first reaction when I saw a snake roadside. My diagnosis from afar was that this one was suffering from overexposure to the sun. But I didn't verify that with a closeup look.

At one point today I had a flashback to a conversation a couple of months ago with a close friend. He was telling me about an MRI he had for his knee. "With all the noise and having half my body in the enclosure, I felt claustrophobic," he said.

"Lucky it wasn't your head being examined," I replied, "because then your entire body would be in the enclosure."

"I couldn't do it," was his reply.

I hate those words, but I said nothing. At age 73 when I started to run across the USA, I was far from sure I could do it. Not until I reached 500 miles did I begin to feel confident.

If after USA someone would have said to me, "Now you've got to run across the other 38 states," again I would have been short on confidence. But never without trying first would I say, "I couldn't do it."

Now that I'm getting close to finishing all 50 states, and now after running thousands of miles, the gospel I preach is: Maybe you think you can't do it, but you probably can if you try and if you really want to do it.

A few passing thoughts in my closing miles of the day:

- Can this be New York, I asked, as a guy in pickup went by and I saw a rifle hanging across the back window of his truck. Smacks more of Wyoming or Montana.

- Must admit that some of the local towns have interesting names: Panama, Dunkirk, Barcelona.

- How long has it been, how many states has it been since I was offered help or a ride? Why the neglect? If I were moving fast, I could understand it. But, slow-paced and ancient as I am, why isn't there some concern for me? Was this reflective of East Coast indifference? Not that I wanted any help or a ride, but it would be reassuring to see some solicitude, some Christian charity.

After finishing our 14.1-mile day, and well aware of how our reconnaissance this morning paid off, we scouted the remaining part of our route to the finish at Lake Erie. Seeing a flat road with a wide shoulder was downright comforting.

Equally comforting was discovering Camp Chautauqua on the shores of Lake Chautauqua. This was a first-class camping resort with 300 spaces, a country store, tennis court, boating facilities and other amenities. Settling in here for the night was painless.

DAY TWO. Last night we stepped into a world I never knew existed. We discovered the Chautauqua Institution, which was located practically adjacent to our campground.

Seeing the lakeside setting, my first reaction was that I was looking at a plushy summer resort. On inquiry I found out that a lot of cultural melting was going on here over a nine-week period extending from late June through late August.

Checking out the calendar of events, I learned that this cultural center includes a theater company, an opera company, a symphony orchestra, and a lecture series. I saw that just in the course of one day a person could listen to a symphony orchestra, attend a lecture, see a live theater performance or be entertained by some name performer. This summer Carol Channing, Rich Little, Willie Nelson, Kenny Rogers, Natalie Cole and Roger Whitaker all made appearances.

I didn't get a chance to check out any of the many accommodations (inns, hotels, guest houses, condominiums) on the Institution grounds or any of the wide array of recreational facilities (golf, tennis, swimming, boating, biking). It was evident that the place was loaded with both quality lodging and good recreational facilities.

My impression, on leaving, was that if a person wanted to be in a setting where he was surrounded with recreational and cultural offerings, this place was unbeatable. Nine weeks of immersion here should equate to a semester in college – yeah, and probably cost as much. The Chautauqua Institution was the most interesting place along our New York routing.

This was somewhat of a dull day on the road. We'd driven the entire route yesterday, so I knew what would unfold along the way. Fact is, I knew little would unfold since there were no special sights along the way today.

I also knew that what I did *not* see was as interesting as what I did see. For one thing, I knew our route was close to Amish Country, but visually we had no evidence of that.

I also knew that Chautauqua County was noted for its Concord grapes, first planted here in 1818, which are used in wines, jellies and juice. It was these Concord grapes that attracted Dr. Charles Welch to the area in 1897.

Anybody who drinks Welch's grape juice knows that the doctor came to the right place. Even though grape production is one of the mainstays of the local economy, I saw not a single vineyard along the way.

What the hell's this, I asked myself when I felt a sharp pain under my right rib cage upon starting this morning? My first reaction was that it would go away in a short while.

Wrong. It stayed with me all day, dimming my enjoyment and causing some concern. When day was done, I knew no more about it than I did at the start.

Philosophically I handled it by saying, It's been a long time since I've run wounded. This will be good for building character.

Thankfully, the road was kind today – flat, comfortable breakdown lane and only moderate traffic. Highway 394, going through the towns of Maryville and Westfield, was a straight shot to Lake Erie. While knowing the route as a result of yesterday's scouting took some luster off the run, it also made the day relaxing in that I knew exactly where I was at all times, how far I had to go and what was coming.

The weather was not as kind as the road. Much of last night we were on the fringes of a severe storm. We could see lightning in the distance, and we heard the thunder.

Traces of this weather were with us when I started under rainy and windy conditions. About a third of the way through our day the rain ceased, but it remained windy and chilly, and the sun never made an appearance.

I did manage to take notice of a few sights along our 12.8-mile route. Going past a cemetery, I did a double take when I saw one of the most unusual tombstones I've ever seen.

It was made of an exquisite marble, global in shape and about four feet in diameter. The double take was necessary to confirm it was a tombstone.

As I saw the "For Sale" signs, I pondered, Why were so many lake waterfront homes for sale? Never did get an answer.

Good cost of living index here, I decided, after seeing the local farmers selling strawberries for $2.49 a basket, whereas in New Jersey the going rate was $1.99.

Couldn't help but admire the many majestic trees along the route.

Crossing a bridge, I silently praised the engineer who had the foresight to put a sidewalk across it. Daring to look over the edge (with age, I've become a coward at heights!), I saw that the drop into the gorge was at least 100 feet.

Foot travel versus car travel: I appreciate a sidewalk, I see a gorge and landmarks; a driver is oblivious to both.

Our passage took us through two towns, Mayville and Westfield.

Both were small (Mayville, 1700; Westfield, 3400) and there was nothing outstanding about either.

On the southern edge of Mayville I did see a number of luxury homes, all of distinctively different design. A photographer would have a ball going through this town and photographing the many differently designed and attractive homes.

A couple of brushes with history in Mayville. One was the home of Judge A. W. Tourge – soldier, author and ambassador to France from 1881 to 1900.

The other touch of history was the Holland Land Company vault, built in 1810. About the size of a single-car garage and used to store the company's records, it was constructed of granite blocks.

Without windows it did have a wooden door made of planks, In my opinion the vault was only as strong as the door, and it appeared vulnerable.

On my journey through Mayville I saw signs advertising a concert in the park on June 26 (good Lord, that's today!) and featuring – oh, how it pains me to say this – Boy Joy!

In downtown Westfield many of the buildings appeared tired, victims of age and weather. Here I came closest to the Concord grape industry, this when I went past the headquarters of the Welch Grape Company – established, so read the plaque, in 1869.

The most recognizable building in town was the First Presbyterian Church, founded in 1824. A three-story building with a gigantic steeple, it was located on the edge of a city park.

The local library of Corinthian design, elaborate for such a small community, spoke eloquently of the community's concern with culture.

Along the way today my mind tumbled with thoughts, which is generally the prevailing mode when I am on the road. Many thoughts. Three that I remembered dealt with something I'd read, an incident on an aircraft carrier and thoughts on suicide.

I recalled something I'd once read, but I could not recall who wrote it. The essence of what he said was that every day a person should hear a song, read a good poem, see a fine picture and try to speak a few reasonable words.

I could go along with that. After all, the guy did not call for dancing!

The aircraft carrier recollection was of a World War II scene in a ready room (the briefing and relaxing room aboard the carrier reserved exclusively for officers with flight status). The pilots had just returned from missions, and the room was filled with excitement, enthusiasm and loud conversation as they talked about their flights.

The squadron commander entered the room and announced, "We've just received a telegram from Admiral Halsey. It reads, "Congratulations to the two-fisted pilot who dived fearlessly into a group of planes and shot down two of the enemy."

All the pilots turned to the pilot who'd done the shooting, and one said, "Well, tell us more."

"Cheez, it all happened so fast," he said. "I saw those planes down there. I wasn't sure if they were Japs or if they were ours, but I just dove in among them and started firing."

Instantly the room went silent. Every pilot had picked up on the words, "not sure if they were ours," and every pilot realized that if they had been "one of ours," he could well be dead. The quietness that followed was eerie.

About suicide: The thinking there was ignited when I recalled a conversation last month with a friend close to my age. Like many older folks we do some thinking and talking about death.

We both agreed that life has been kind to us, that we've lead full lives and that we are not fearful of death itself. What we both dread there is the possibility of a long terminal illness that will put a burden on our loved ones, and one that could strip us of our dignity to the point were we are mental marshmallows or bedridden – maybe putrefying or wallowing in our urine and feces, and all the while having no purpose to live.

Where we part company is that if he finds himself near or approaching those circumstances, he will unhesitantly kill himself. I envy him in that, without any feeling of guilt, he will choose suicide as a way of escape.

I wish I could. Time and again I've mulled over why I wouldn't. I think the basic reason is because I feel suicide is self-murder, something that would get me in trouble with God (and the timing would be very bad here since it would be judgment day!).

The only other reason I can conjure up for negating suicide is that it could simply be out of cowardice on my part. I regard suicide to spare loved ones pain, anguish and sorrow as a brave act.

Here I am talking about suicide by a person physically or mentally devastated, a terminally ill person, a person so ravaged by illness that life is meaningless. I am not talking about suicide by an person mentally competent and able-bodied, which is irrational, escapism and unfair to those left behind.

In one way, I thought, this suicide thing is a little bit like combat. You never know how you (or others) will react until the bullets start flying.

At this point I am dealing in theory. Suicide is out either because it's self-murder or because I'm a coward, or maybe because of both.

Would I be so convinced if I found myself in a situation where suicide was the best way out for all? Maybe suicide could be in.

Suicide was the centerpiece for one of the most memorable movie scenes I've ever seen. The movie was "Soylent Green."

In it Edward G. Robinson, an old man failing in both mind and body, decides the time has come for him to exit from life. He goes to the place that the government operates for people of his mind set and condition.

There he lies down in a comfortable setting, and as he is lying there beautiful and serene scenes swirl around the walls and ceiling of the room, and soothing music is in the background. As he's watching and listening to things beautiful, the technology of the time painlessly terminates his life. Why can't our society be that kind?

A bit of a smile when I thought of Dorothy Parker's objection to suicide. It went like this:

> *Razors pain you;*
> *Rivers are damp;*
> *Acids stain you;*
> *And drugs cause cramp.*
> *Guns aren't lawful;*
> *Nooses give;*
> *Gas smells awful;*
> *You might as well live.*

After leaving Westfield, I followed Highway 394, went over the I-90 overpass, and continued on 394 until it intersected with Lake Erie near the Barcelona Harbor Ramp. There I wrapped up what was beginning to be like another day at the office.

Nineteen states done on this trip, two to go – Michigan and Wisconsin. After finishing, we lingered in New York only long enough to take some pictures, then we headed for nearby I-90 and took off for Michigan.

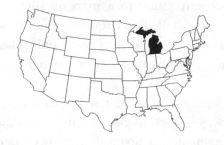

Chapter 20

Michigan

Thumbing My Way Across the State

Dates: *June 29th to July 1st, 1997*
Miles: *40.9*
Route: *Start on Highway 142 at water's edge of Lake Huron at Harbor Beach and follow 142 west to water's edge at Saginaw Bay near Bayport, Michigan's west border.*

DAY ONE. Damn lucky I'm starting Michigan today and not yesterday, I told myself while getting underway. Yesterday I would have had to contend with 656 bicyclists on Highway 142 and headed for Harbor Bay, my starting point.

The riders were participating in the PALM (Peddling Across Lower Michigan) annual bike ride, extending seven days and 300 miles. The unique feature of this ride, as apart from others, is that it's designed for beginners. The youngest rider was 6; the oldest, 83.

Even if these bicyclists were on the road, this would have been a bush-league problem. Major league would be in Iowa contending with the 10,000 riders in RAGBRAI (the Register's Annual Great Bike Ride Across Iowa), covering 464 miles, west to east, from the Missouri River to the Mississippi River, in seven days.

I tried to visualize 10,000 people, all seeking lodging and food, descending on a small Iowa town for the night. Even though most of the riders were tenting, all I could see was chaos and confusion – and a long parade of portable potties rolling across the state for a one-night stand.

I'd never given any study to a map of Michigan until I began planning to run across it. It didn't require more than a cursory look to see that Michigan is divided into two peninsulas, the upper and lower. Among the 50 states it is unique in being divided into two peninsulas.

As I kept looking at the map, it soon became apparent that the lower peninsula was shaped like a mitten. As I studied the situation, comparing the peninsulas, I favored the lower because it seemed more kindly disposed to running, being flat, being more developed and having more facilities (especially campgrounds and markets).

The original route that I selected was across the four-fingers part of the mitten, west to east, from Petosky to Rogers City. Following my standard operating procedure, I contacted two friends to get background information about the state and the route.

Bill Weinstein – a Marine Corps classmate, prominent Detroit attorney and major general in the Marine Corps Reserve – provided some useful information about the state. His letter was a little difficult for me to read since he wrote it on his Marine Corps stationery, the top of which was adorned with a red flag and two white stars of a major general, which necessitated that I had to stand at rigid attention as I held it and read.

My second contact, A.J. Underwood, was a friend of 25 years, an age-class runner and a founder of the Buffalo Chips Running Club in Sacramento. A.J., who had transplanted from Michigan to work for the state of California, said, "You know, if you're looking for the shortest distance across the state, you ought to take a look at The Thumb. My suggestion is that you take Highway 142 which is a little over 40 miles across The Thumb."

A. J. was referring to the part of the mitten-shaped peninsula resembling a thumb. And look at Highway 142 I did, which resulted in the decision to run from the water's edge at Harbor Beach to the water's edge at Bayport.

When we arrived at our starting area in Harbor Beach, I knew from our drive across 142 that the route I'd run was indeed very runnable. I thought it would hold no surprises since we'd become acquainted with it while driving.

We did get one surprise at the start, though. We had driven to the water's edge at the eastern extension of 142 and just as I started running, with Elaine in front of me, a guy in a van came speeding toward us and yelled, "You're on private property! Get out!"

"That's what we're doing," I said

"Well, get moving," he said.

"Look, I'm starting to run across the state and I'm moving as fast as I can," I told him.

Elaine, seeing and hearing all this , slowed the motorhome to the point where I was right behind her. The guy started edging his van toward us.

Again he yelled, "You're on private property. Private property. Get your ass outta here!"

"Are you the police?" I replied.

"No, I'm the shift supervisor, and I'm telling you to get off private property," he blustered.

I looked around, expecting to see a plant in operation and a number of cars belonging to workers. The only car I saw was his, and I concluded he must be supervising himself.

He tailgated us during our entire quarter-mile exit and a couple more times yelled, "Private property. Get outta here" He was typical of the type that has a private's authority and responsibility, and exercises it with Napoleonic zeal.

The town of Harbor Beach was adjacent to the plant area. I asked the first person I saw there about the plant.

"Oh, it's the Star Chemical Company," he said, "but I don't know what they make."

The only business that appeared to be open this Sunday morning was Mom's Restaurant. The downtown section of three blocks or so consisted of a number of small store fronts and of nothing particularly noteworthy.

Once out of town I ran on a four-foot gravel shoulder, remindful of Iowa where I ran on a similar gravel surface across the entire state. I would have preferred the pavement, but the fog line came to the very edge of the paved surface and that meant I'd have to run on the road itself.

This would be safe with approaching cars because I could see them and then jump to the gravel. But it would be dangerous because of cars behind me passing another car and entering the lane where I would be running.

The gravel, with all the slipping and sliding it caused, was somewhat unkind to my legs. The problem was accentuated often because the Highway Department was overly generous in spots with its spreading of gravel on the shoulder, and the deep bed of gravel was hard to negotiate.

With a faint attempt at humor, I could say the going was rocky. At least, though, it was safe.

As I went along, I found myself recognizing that here and now would be a good time to have a running friend alongside of me for conversation. With nothing but agriculture on both sides of the road, the setting was humdrum.

Oh, there were a few sights. The first was when, seeing a side view, I asked myself, Why does this guy have a bathtub leaning against the side of his house?

When I arrived for a frontal view, I saw that the tub housed a statute of the Blessed Virgin Mary holding the infant Jesus. With that kind of a setting, could this guy be related to Andy Warhol?

The sight of a mailbox with the name Michener on it brought to mind a post-World War II experience. I was in a bookstore and saw a book, *Tales of the South Pacific*, by James A. Michener.

In the 21st Marines I'd served with a Captain James A. Michener, who before the war had been a newspaper reporter. Somewhat naturally my first reaction on seeing the book was, Jim's used his South Pacific experiences to write a book. False assumption, I soon learned when reading about the author on the book's jacket.

At one point I stopped to study a field planted with lettuce – thousands and thousands of heads. The stuff is selling for almost $2 a head, and this field is worth a fortune.

Then I fell to wondering just how much of that $2 does the farmer get? How many middlemen (wholesaler, market, etc.) are between him and the buyer?

One sight today proved that, at least to a small degree, trust still prevails in America. I passed a roadside stand where apples were for sale. It was unattended and a sign read, "Three-pound bag, $1.50. Half a bushel, $6.50. Please leave money in box or come to the house."

I performed one heroic act today. This happened when, just ahead, I saw something on the road.

Arriving on the scene, I saw a frog which seemed immobilized because of too much sun exposure. I picked him up and carried him to the nearby grass.

Then as I got a few steps down the road, I realized he could use more help to resurrect so I returned, poured water on him and saw signs of some revival. For sure that guy should be glad I was out here and not in church this Sunday.

There have been times, fleeting moments, in my life when I've thought I've been protected by a guardian angel or a sixth sense. One of those moments happened today when I was running on the gravel.

A red pickup, approaching from my rear, passed another car, cut over the fog line and occupied the two-foot bike lane. Had I been exercising my option of running in that bike lane, he would have hamburgered me.

What mostly got me through this day was doing a lot of thinking. Some unknown wag once said, "Sometimes I sits and thinks, and sometimes I just sits."

I could paraphrase that to, Sometimes I runs and thinks, and sometimes I just thinks. Today seemed like one of those days.

All this thinking ignited when I remembered this was Sunday, the day when I customarily take time out to dwell on God and things spiritual. As I started to do so, I was soon immersed in some deep self-exploration when I asked myself, Just what do I believe?

What is my credo – as apart from the Credo (both Nicene and Apostles') of the Catholic church I've recited so many times (at one stage in my life, I could rattle off the Credo in Latin). My body was in motion, but my mind was far removed from running as I tried to frame what I believed.

Groping for a beginning, I tried to recall something I'd read in the distant past. My recollection was that Thomas Jefferson or Thomas Paine had said it, but I was unsure of that. I was also fuzzy about the exact words, but the thrust of what was said was still very clear.

Jefferson, Paine or whoever had said, speaking of things spiritual, that he could accept only what he could arrive at by his own thinking, by his own reasoning. Somewhat diametrically opposed to a Mohandas "Mahatma" Gandhi utterance, "Religion is not what is grasped by the brain, but a heart grasp."

I'm not sure what Gandhi meant by a "heart grasp", but my observation is that for the most part religion is what a person inherits by nature of birth. In most cases, it comes from parents or from country, just like language is inherited by nature of birth.

So I was back to Jefferson, Paine or whoever. I did recall that Paine once said, "My mind is my church."

My mind, my thinking, my reasoning – that sounded like a good starting point for me. Using such, what credo could I form?

Oh boy, no sooner than thinking that did I realize I was speaking what most if not all clerics would consider heresy. I was rejecting faith.

I kicked that around for a while and decided that faith is to religion as hearsay is to law. Ipso facto, disregard faith.

Back to ground zero: Just what is my credo based on thinking/reasoning, taking nothing on faith? Instantly as I began this self-exploration, I realized I was in trouble because of the limited capabilities of my mind. Besides, this type of thinking was tough.

So much easier to take it all on faith. No wonder so many do.

Damn it, I'm not going to surrender. I'll try to fight this thing through. On with the credo.

1. I believe in God. Accepted not on faith, but from the orderliness of the world, the science of the universe. There has to be a reason for the profound difference between man and the animal kingdom, and that reason has to be God. About the nature of God, I know only that He is all-powerful, omnipotent. I now think that the catechism line "Man is made in the image and likeness of God" is the most egoistic utterance I've ever heard and borders on blasphemy. Another reason I believe in God is that without Him man's existence would be meaningless. Maybe that's why Voltaire said, "If God did not exist, it would be necessary to invent Him."

2. It follows that if God does exist, we are God's creatures.

3. If we are God's creatures, God put us here for a purpose. Surely, we are not here for His amusement or as His toys, for such He does not need.

4. Granting that God does exist, He has from the very beginning of time. "In the beginning was the Word and the Word is God" – that I buy. It is a sine qua non of God existing. A corollary is that God will always exist. That so, it seems reasonable, then, that if God created people, His grand design called for at least

some of them to share eternity with Him. Thus I believe in ever-lasting life.

5. The key question that follows would be, How does He choose the "some"? Well, in the first place, God being God, being all-just, it would follow that every person born would have an equal opportunity to be included in the some. That's a simple premise, but if it is subscribed to the conclusion is that there is no one true religion, which is something Robert Burton, himself a clergyman, said many years ago: "One religion is as true as another." To put it another way, I believe every religion offers an equal opportunity for its believers to be included in the some. Beyond that I believe a person has an equal oppor-tunity even if he subscribes to no religion. I just can't believe that any of the 17 million Jews, two billion Christians, one billion Moslems or any others have an inside track. The playing field is level for every person ever created.

6. The key, it would seem, to whether or not we will be included in the some is how we live our lives, what we do with the life God has given us. The question here then becomes what code of conduct by God's standards applies to all people, regardless of their religious beliefs or lack of such – or perhaps to their adherence of such. I believe that each person is responsible to God for living by a code of conduct.

7. That transcends to, What code of conduct? Is it the same for all people, in all nations? At first utterance, that sounds ridiculous, all people/all nations. But in basic tenets I am not sure it is. To me it seems reasonable that condemnation of murder/rape/ robbery should be cardinal to any code of conduct. The only code of conduct I know anything about is the Ten Commandants. The problem with this code is that in some instances, it has been messed up with priestly or ecclesiastical interpretations. As but once instance, sixth commandant, adultery – interpreted to church doctrines on divorce, birth control, abortion, at least in the Catholic church. (Interesting to note here that Judaism recognizes divorce as a catastrophe that is bound to happen and it provides a means to dissolve such marriages. Speaking of Judaism, there's an old saying, "It's tough to be a Jew." Sort of understandable considering their "code" has 613 commands.)

Oh hell, I caught myself thinking, I'm going around in circles. Focus on code of conduct. What is my code of conduct? Just how much can I pinpoint it? Well, let's see:

I certainly believe in worship of God.

I positively believe murder, rape, robbery, incest are wrong.

I believe that matters pertaining to marriage and sex are matters of individual conscience, including divorce and birth control.

I believe we should treat other people like we would like to be treated.

I believe each person is entitled to his own religious beliefs but in exercising them he should not interfere with others.

I've come to the point where I no longer believe the Catholic precepts that missing church is sinful, that eating meat on forbidden Fridays is sinful, that divorce is sinful, that confession is necessary for God's forgiveness.

If only because we would have anarchy without such, I believe that a system of justice is indispensable with full equity and responsibility for everyone. A corollary of this is that a person is responsible for his actions.

Those were the thoughts I spoke into my cassette recorder as I went down the road. Even though they are wobbly in spots, even though there's some lack of coherence, even though my reasoning may be faulty, I have not edited them because that would result in a distorted view of my mental meanderings as I went down the road.

Our game plan today had been that I'd run 16.5 miles, but that got sabotaged by the time I reached 15.4 miles and a severe lightning and thunder storm descended on us. We have an inviolate rule: no running during lightning.

The nearest camping after we finished was a KOA in Port Austin, at the northern tip of The Thumb, which was a 20-mile drive. We settled in there for a comfortable night.

Looking back on the day, I assessed it as an easy running day, albeit the gravel shoulder was a bit of a nuisance. On the plus side my bruised heel that had bothered me throughout New York emitted no distress signals. The weather – mid-70s, slight wind, clouds polka-doting the sky – was kind until the storm struck.

DAY TWO. The most pleasurable aspect of our 20-mile drive from the

KOA Kampground near Port Austin to the start of our second day in Michigan was that the drive was along a road we'd not be running on and thus not repeating. This road was Highway 53 that bisected The Thumb in a north-south direction.

On the map, Highway 53 was a red-lined road, whereas 142 was black-lined. But in actuality the two roads were quite similar even to the point of being lined on both sides with agriculture.

On Highway 142 I started about two miles east of Bad Axe and had gone only a mile or so when a police vehicle pulled up behind me. The vehicle's door emblem told me the officer was from the Huron sheriff's department.

I was impressed with the size of the officer when he stepped out of the car. He was about as big as the typical Michigan State tackle.

A famous psychologist, William Morgan, once observed that we are built for fight or flight. He fight, me flight, I thought.

Sergeant Gary Polega greeted me with these words: "Just checking on how you're doing out here."

"Doing okay," I said, "but I'd be better if this gravel were paved."

"How far are you running?" he asked.

After I recited my story, I said, "I bet you don't see many old guys like me out here doing this."

"Well, to tell the truth, that's right," he replied. "I've been with the department 22 years, and you're a first."

"Twenty-two years," I said. "You must like the job."

"Love the job," he told me. "How can I complain, got my own car and everything. Does get kind of rough out here, though, some days in winter. Like when it gets as cold as 20 degrees below zero."

I shivered at the thought, then curious I asked, "Can you tell me how Bad Axe got its name?"

"Yeah," he said, "some old feller found an axe lying in the area and, apparently, you know, it was a real old axe. I think it was busted or something, so they decided to call it 'Bad Axe' and it stuck."

After the sergeant drove off, I tried to recall how long it had been since a police officer, highway patrol or sheriff, had stopped to check on me. Which state was it? Must have been quite a while ago because I didn't have the faintest recollection.

I knew that the city of Bad Axe would be the most variation today from the agriculture setting, so I resolved to sashay through it slowly and to take a good look around. Bad Axe was typical of a small city of 3500 – but because I was coming out of the agriculture setting that had engulfed me, it appeared metropolitan. I blushed to admit that my best remembrance of the place was Murphy's Bakery, with apple fritters par excellence, as Elaine could also testify.

While leisurely going through town, I saw a turtle-designed lamp in a store window and took time out to buy it as a birthday present for my son-in-law Dan Phillips, who collects turtle paraphernalia. Now the challenge is to see if we can get it home without breaking it.

I did take note of two different signs, one informing me that Bad Axe is the county seat of Huron County and the other that it's the site of the Huron County Fair. I also noted that all the residences in Bad Axe were modest – nothing elaborate, nothing shabby.

Ever the tourist, I took a picture of the downtown section where the local theater was showing "Batman and Robin." Doing so, I registered a bit of surprise at seeing a first-run feature playing here so soon after release.

Biggest business in town seemed to be the John Deere dealership. It appeared to have at least one of every piece of farm equipment that Deere makes. As I looked at all this stuff, I thought, if I could take time out for a tutorial on each piece of equipment here, learning how it operates and what its purpose is, I'd come away with a pretty good understanding of farming operations.

A sign told me the place was owned by a guy named Gettell. He must be Daddy Big Bucks in these parts, I concluded, because since starting at Harbor Beach I'd now seen this dealership and three General Motors dealerships owned by him.

The name Gettell brought back memories of days at University of California at Berkeley. There I took a course in political theory from a professor named Gettell.

He was unusual in that he was a full professor, despite having only a master's degree (from Amherst) and not a Ph.D. I remembered that he never looked at any notes during his lectures, and he was never dull.

I had the privilege of taking an individual honors reading course from him. Whenever we met to discuss the books I'd read, I was awed with his knowledge and with what a gracious gentleman he was.

At one of the first pit stops today Elaine reported that on their CB radios the truckers were talking about the old guy out on the road running for a Mexican cause. Huh? What was I missing in this equation?

One thing this jaunt across Michigan was doing for me, I told myself, was to correct my lopsided, stereotyped view of the state. Previously when Michigan came to mind, I thought in terms of automobile manufacturing and assembly lines.

Now I realized that the state is rich in agriculture and recreational areas. Here was another state whose park facilities, state and county, were far superior to California's. Here, as I went along, I was seeing fields of soy beans, sugar beats, wheat , corn, lettuce – and not automobile plants.

As in so many other farm settings, I passed by a farm that had a sign with the owner's name – in this case Ray Herber and sons. Which set me to thinking: Nice to see the farm will stay in the family, passed on to the sons.

But my question was, What happens when there is a daughter or daughters in the family? I've never seen a sign with "& Daughters" on it.

Are they always left out in the cold? After mulling that, another thought: Boy, that observation should make brownie points with NOW!

A dozen or so miles into the day I was treated to a second variation from the farm scene when I came to Elkton. I had a hard time equating what I saw there to the nearly 1000 population the town sign proclaimed.

The most imposing edifices in Elkton were 20 huge grain silos. Nearby was a water tower on which some humorist had painted a happy face. That for me was a first, so out came the trusty Olympus for a photo.

The poster-sized menu outside of Giovanni's Family Restaurant caught my eye: pork stir fry, Polish walleye, hamburger stroganoff, goulash. Four good reasons to make the place off limits to me.

One enjoyable feature of going through Elkton was enjoying the shade provided by the town's many trees. Got me to thinking that this Michigan route is a contrast to the New England states where I was always surrounded by trees. Here they are rare, and ditto with the mountains that were so prevalent in New England.

I did a considerable amount of reflecting while on the road today. Sort of a potpourri of thoughts rather than focusing on anything.

I remembered back to a few days ago when I commented on an acquaintance saying, "I couldn't do that." I reflected on how much fun in life Elaine and I would have missed if I'd taken that attitude when I first thought of running across the USA.

Related to that, I should have added something I read recently: "The man who misses all the fun is the one who says it can't be done."

One of the many lessons I've learned from being on the road is the truth of Sir James Barrie's words, "Life is a long lesson in humility." As the years of life mount, I am more impressed with what I don't know than with what I do know.

An example, I go down the road and see many varieties of trees, but at best I can identify only 20 percent of them. Likewise with geological formations, but here the identification percentage drops to five percent.

Weather is still a mystery; I even have trouble with cirrus and cumulus clouds. Meet someone speaking a foreign language (like the Mexican guys in New Mexico when I wanted directions or the Mexican guy in North Dakota who stopped me on a freeway exit to ask for information), and I'm tongue-tied. I read the elevation from the little altimeter on the motorhome dashboard and I haven't the foggiest idea of how it works.

The knowledge explosion overwhelms me. Sometimes borders on depressing to think about how much I don't know. "A long lesson in humility" – right on, Sir James!

Another thing I've come to recognize from my meandering and meditating on the road is that one key to happiness it for a person to find one thing he's good at, one thing he likes, then do it, concentrate on it, revel in it. Maybe the person's forte is a sport, maybe it's making or building things, maybe it's cars or something mechanical, or maybe it's art or books or collection – maybe any one of dozens of things.

The point is that a person immersed in something he enjoys, possibly excels, is most likely to find happiness just in doing it. God knows that Elaine and I have found a lot of happiness with such a simple thing as being out here on the road and coming to understand and appreciate this vast land with all its beauty and natural resources.

This was another one of those days when, from a distance of one mile, I could see Elaine parked ahead for a pit stop, and each time I saw her it seemed I had a tough time reigning her in. I felt infernally slow. But it was nice to have a target to zero in on.

For her part Elaine, who was raised on a farm in Idaho, was enjoying the setting, somewhat remindful of her upbringing. The moderate traffic and the gravel shoulder that accommodated her parking and my running eased the going for both of us.

She did complain, though, of the problem she had with Rebel and Brudder on one of their walks. The boys sniffed a dead deer and, locating it, tried to indulge in a venison binge.

Elaine had other ideas. "It took all the strength I had pulling on the leashes to dissuade them," she reported.

As almost a re-run of yesterday our plan to cover 16.5 miles was jettisoned when a vicious storm hit the area about the time I'd logged 15.5 miles. Lightning was striking frighteningly close by the time I got into the motorhome.

One bolt hit so close that both Elaine and I thought we could reach out and touch it. The thunder was causing the dogs to panic. Scared and unable to find a place to hide in the motorhome, they practically clung to us.

The rain was so torrential that at times visibility in front of the motorhome was not much beyond the hood. We decided to drive slowly and cautiously up the west coast of The Thumb on Highway 25 and to stay at one of the state parks or at a county park located on the coast of Saginaw Bay.

As we drove northward, the rainstorm continued to be so severe that on a couple of occasions when we could find a safe parking area, we pulled roadside and parked a few moments. All the while the road was getting covered with more and more water, and the muddy shoulders invited disaster.

Our plan to stay overnight in one of the three parks failed. One had a sign, "Campground full," and the other two were swamped with water. Even if we could locate an empty spot in either of these two, the motorhome would be surrounded by water and any electrical connection would be dangerous.

We decided that our best bet was to drive to the KOA near Port Austin where we had stayed last night. We both remembered it as being on high ground and thus protected from flooding. Arriving at the KOA after a 35-mile drive, not only did we find the RV park relatively dry but also we learned that the brunt of the storm had passed to the west of the campground.

We were so concerned with getting safely located in the RV park that we took no note of the town of Port Austin, located on the northern tip of The Thumb. Settling in for the night, we derived ecstatic pleasure from the simple relief of people, beasts and vehicle having escaped the storm and now being safely and comfortably located in the RV park. As we used to say in my altar boy days, Deo gratias.

DAY THREE. Always a great feeling, as I experienced during our 30-mile drive to the start today, to know that by the end of the day I will have finished another state. But, in truth, the feeling was not as satisfying on this as it had been previous summers.

The reason was simple: On USA I'd averaged 26 miles a day; on the states west of the Mississippi, 21 miles a day; now on the states east of the Mississippi, only 17 a day. The challenge was considerably less this year, and the satisfaction decreased proportionately.

Yet, almost conversely, just being out here and mobile at 80, was a source of some satisfaction. I never cease to be astounded over living 80 years.

When I was 40, 50, 60, I never foresaw such longevity in my future. Between 60 and 80 I've seen so many friends die that I've often wondered, why they and not me, often recalled the biblical passage "one will be taken" and why that one and not me.

Different feelings with different deaths – when the person is older, I feel I still have a few years, some relaxation sets in; when the person is younger, I feel I've overlived my time, I'm about due to step over the Great Divide.

In between these two viewpoints lies one of the greatest joys and benefits of running. As much as anything else it has helped me to enjoy the sensation of just being alive.

Our biggest apprehension on getting underway this morning was the weather. All through the night we were in a moderate rain.

The fear was another storm today. So far in Michigan we were batting two for two: two days and two storms.

We had only nine miles to go to finish, and the only deterrent to that would be a violent storm. With only a light rain as we started on Highway 142, we felt fortunate and grateful.

Once again, as with the previous two days, we were in an agriculture setting. This inspired Elaine to revert to her childhood days on an Idaho farm because when she saw a cultivated field with at least 300 seagulls on it, she recited this childhood verse.

> *One for the magpie.*
> *One for the crow,*
> *One for the blackbird,*
> *and One to grow.*

All new stuff to a city boy like me. For sure I'd not seen it in any classical literature!

The only time I got out of the farm setting during the entire 8.8-mile day was during the passage through the small town of Pigeon, inescapable inasmuch as Highway 142 bisects the town.

Pigeon appeared to have sufficient stores to accommodate the daily needs of the local citizenry, but nothing more than that. I saw no distinctive or distinguishable landmarks or buildings. The local newspaper, The *Pigeon Tribune*, which I picked up out of curiosity, could be read in its entirety in five minutes.

The running day was pretty much routine up until the last 1.5 miles. I plodded along, two pit stops on the way, just covering the miles, always with an eye on the sky and the weather.

About the time I had 1.5 miles left, the skies erupted with a fury – rain, lightning, thunder. Elaine was already at the finish, waiting for me, and besides with such a short distance left, I had no choice but to ignore our inviolate rule and run during the lightning.

Soaked, fighting a headwind and squishing through an inch or two of water on the road, I was glad to come upon Highway 25, the north-south road on the west side of The Thumb that signaled the finish was near. Crossing 25, I got onto an unnamed road that led to Saginaw Bay and the finish.

When I had 500 yards to go and could see Elaine parked ahead, I became aware of a weird phenomenon: I was suddenly out of the rain and into a dry area. It was as if I'd run through a curtain, rain on one side and dry on the other.

"You look soaked," Elaine announced when I arrived at the finish. "In fact, you look almost drowned."

"Which leaves me wondering, how come you and the dogs are so dry?" I replied.

"Why shouldn't we be?" she said. "We haven't had a drop of rain here."

During the day I made the miles go by faster by indulging in my usual mental gymnastics as I went down the road. I dwelled a few moments on all the ballyhoo back in the John F. Kennedy administration about a 50-mile hike.

All the hoopla started when General David M. Shoup, then commandant of the Marine Corps, sent President Kennedy a Teddy Roosevelt document about some physical tests. Shoup was surprised when JFK responded by saying, in effect, why don't you try these tests on some Marines?

The result was that some officers were randomly selected and given marching orders: Walk 50 miles in no more than three days, with actual walking time and rest stops limited to 20 hours. Upon reaching the final half-mile, the officers were to double-time (meaning simply to jog) 200 yards, rest for 30 seconds, then double-time for 300 yards, rest a minute and wind up with a 200-yard dash to the finish line.

How our perspectives change. Back then, at age 46 and not yet into distance running, I considered those marching orders a strenuous and challenging physical test.

Now, after 34 years as a distance runner, I consider them creampuff stuff. Why? Good Lord, at age 50 Ted Corbitt, ran (that's faster than "double-time") 50 miles in five hours, 34 minutes.

Ted Corbitt, now there's a story few Americans know about. A black guy who did his training on the streets of New York City and ran phenomenal times for 50 and 100 miles.

Good enough marathoner, too, to be on the USA Olympic team. Quiet-spoken, modest, courteous, superb athlete. Great as he was, it would still be a safe bet today that not more than one out of 50 high school or college students could identify him.

Not only Corbitt but other older runners made the Shoup/Roosevelt fitness test look ridiculous. Frans Pauwel at age 60 covered 50 miles in six hours, 24 minutes, and a number of runners in their 70s (including George Billingsley with whom I sometimes run) have run 50 miles in the eight-hour range. Once spooked by the distance, I have run 15 races of 50 miles – including 6:38 at age 55 and 7:19 at age 64.

Yeah, one of the many things I've learned as a runner was all that media hype about 50 miles back in the JFK area was – how did Shakespeare put it? – "full of sound and fury signifying nothing." More succinctly, as my Uncle Paul would have said, "Bushwa."

Chilled at one point today, I thought back to World War II and the time I spent in MOB 4 Hospital in Auckland, New Zealand, when malaria hit me for the first time. Some moments, even though wrapped in four blankets, I'd be chilling and chattering; other moments my body felt on fire.

Still vivid in my mind is what happened one night in our ward there. About 40 of us were in the ward – some with malaria, some with elephantiasis, one guy blinded, another with his guts blasted out, a guy with both legs cut off when he parachuted and a Japanese pilot in a Zero cut off his legs with the plane's propeller. Forty guys in trouble.

The happening occurred one night when we were all listening to a radio program blaring in the ward. A long-beaked comedian cracking jokes had all the guys laughing until tears rolled down their cheeks. This laugh-happy mug was Bob Hope.

A husky-throated woman sang "Moonlight Becomes You So," and most of the guys were misty eyed, pains and worries momentarily set aside. Next Hope introduced "a fat little man who sings," and again the focus, at least momentarily, was on him and not on troubles. That night, that experience is why for me Bob Hope, Dinah Shore, and Bing Crosby will never die.

After taking our usual finish pictures, this time with Saginaw Bay in the background, we headed north toward Gaylord where we had mail waiting – a package from Keokee Publishing Company that contained page proofs of our forthcoming book *Go East Old Man*. Our next major task was to proofread this manuscript and to return it to Keokee ASAP.

Having the mail arrive at Gaylord was based on our original plan to run west to east, from Petosky to Rogers City. Since Gaylord put us so far north, we decided to continue north, cross the Mackinac Bridge, and travel across the Upper Peninsula of Michigan to reach Wisconsin, our next state. Another reason for routing this way was that it avoided the southern route and its metropolitan areas, particularly Detroit.

The drive over the Mackinac Bridge turned out to be the most exciting (and scary) part of our day. The weather was miserable, the wind ferocious, visibility limited, and traffic was restricted to 20 miles per hour. Vehicles were bumper to bumper, and we were lucky enough to be snuggled behind a semi that sheltered us to some degree from the wind.

The Mackinac Bridge is the longest suspension bridge in the world with 7400 feet of four-lane roadway suspended over the Straits of Mackinac. The total length of the bridge, including its approaches, is approximately five miles. To us this day the distance across "Big Mac" seemed more like 15 miles.

From this gateway to the Upper Peninsula, Mackinac Island with its renowned Grand Hotel, is visible. But we weren't looking. All across the bridge our eyes were fixed on that friendly semi just ahead of us.

This bridge crossing was one of the very few times in our lives that Elaine and I appreciated being caught in bumper-to-bumper traffic. It deterred some reckless type from exceeding the 20-MPH speed limit and thus endangering other drivers.

The satisfaction of finishing Michigan was minor compared to that felt after getting safely across the bridge. Elaine, who has always harbored a hankering to drive a semi, handled the motorhome masterfully. Much more of that and she'll be joining the teamsters' union.

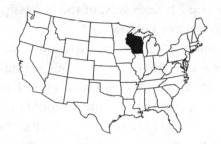

Chapter 21

Wisconsin

Swan Song for the Motorhome

Dates: *July 6th and 7th, 1997*
Miles: *27.7*
Route: *Start at east border of Wisconsin, Lake Michigan, at Algoma, and take Highway 54 west to its junction with Highway 1. Then follow Highway 1 and Algoma/Scottwood/Nicholet to reach waters of Green Bay, the west border of Wisconsin.*

DAY ONE. July 4th for us the past six years that we've been on the road has been more grimace than grin. Because of the holiday we've usually been caught in a rat race trying to find an overnight home for the motorhome. The routine has been seeing a "Park full" sign, then scouting around until we found a place to stay.

When we arrived at Green Bay late afternoon on July 2nd, that was the scenario we expected to see unfold. Instead, arriving at the Brown County Fairgrounds with its RV park, we found the park only 10-percent occupied. "Can this be for real?" was our reaction.

The second surprise: This facility was better than 80 percent of the RV parks – full hookups (electrical, water, sewer), beautiful setting (lawns and shady trees) on the banks of the Fox River, and removed from any major highway. The Fox River took on added meaning when I remembered that slightly over 300 years ago the explorers Father Jacques Marquette and Louis Joliet had traveled it.

We were lucky to be in such surroundings because we had work to do, reading the page proofs of *Go East Old Man* (chronicling our adventures across the 22 states west of the Mississippi) and returning the corrections to Keokee Publishing.

Over dinner July 2nd Elaine and I decided on our strategy for doing the proofreading. The essence of our planning was that we'd take three days off from the road and complete the project by proofing 100 pages a day. That schedule would allow Elaine time to walk her dogs and do other chores, for me to jog three miles a day to stay tuned, and for the two of us to do some sightseeing in Green Bay.

Sightseeing, I found the downtown section of Green Bay, a city with a population of 67,000 remindful of Sacramento, California, where I lived back in the days when it had a similar population. A pleasant small-city atmosphere radiating much civic pride.

Being loyal 49er fans, Elaine and I made a pilgrimage to Lambeau Field Stadium to see the site where in recent years our beloved Niners have been martyred by the Packers. The Packer Hall of Fame is across from Lambeau Field, but having no desire to see Super Bowl trophies we had hoped for the 49ers to win, we stayed away. All the while when on this Packer turf and being aware of the rashness of Packer fans (Example: dissatisfied with their coach, Dan Devine, they shot his dog!), we kept our 49er affiliation a secret.

For a small city Green Bay was loaded with tourist attractions. We wanted to visit the National Railway Museum and see the private railway car used by General Eisenhower in World War II, but parking the motorhome and leaving the dogs was unmanageable.

By chance, while driving around on July 4th we were lucky enough to see some of the Cardboard Regatta Race on the Fox River. All we knew about the event was that boats were made out of cardboard and raced a specified distance.

The race was more survival than speed because many of the boats sank on their way. The crowd got many laughs watching the frantic efforts and antics of the boaters trying to stay afloat.

After a three-day vacation, gearing up for our first day across Wisconsin was as tough as returning to work on a Monday after a fun weekend. Look, I told myself in a pep talk, you're damn lucky to have escaped Michigan unscathed and just to be here to run. So get on with it.

I was referring to the fact that when we left Michigan, we had a choice of departing to the north via the upper peninsula or going southward on the lower peninsula. We went north. Had we gone south, we would have been smack in the middle of a storm and tornado that killed eight people.

Looking for a short route across the state, we focused on the Door Peninsula. We decided to scout a route that went west to east from the shores of Green Bay to Highway 1, then connecting with Highway 54 that led to Algoma and the shores of Lake Michigan.

We found the 28-mile route along the base of the Door Peninsula easy pickings – almost flat, moderate traffic, wide gravel shoulder. We decided to split the run into two days, 16 miles and 12 miles, and to start at Algoma and run west.

This route had its pluses and minuses. On the plus side the distance was short and technically and geographically across the state. Short as the route was, I could have reduced it by two-thirds by running across the northern part of the peninsula.

On the minus side it was a far throw from the 156-miles route I had originally planned to run, a route recommended by Jeff Roznowski of Wauwatona. Following this route on Highway 11 across southern Wisconsin, I would have seen much more of the state than on the shorter Highway 54 route.

Today's start was rare in that it was in such a beautiful setting, a small park in Algoma on the shores of Lake Michigan. After touching the lake's water, then pausing momentarily to take a look at the adjoining marina, I crossed the sandy beach and got on the Crescent Boardwalk which paralleled the beach embankment with manicured grass and flower beds.

If the Algoma Chamber of Commerce had not told me, I'd never realized the boardwalk was made of recycled plastic. A sign told me that dogs, bicyclists, skaters and roller-bladers were prohibited.

A town of 3500 population, Algoma seemed well-balanced between tourism and industry. There appeared to be a heavy concentration of motels and restaurants, but by the same token Algoma had more than its share of industry (a hardwood company, a mop manufacturer, a net company, a label company, a charter-fishing industry, among others).

The lady I talked with in the Chamber of Commerce told me, "It's too bad you won't be here for our Shanty Days Festival next month. It's a big celebration. We have a parade, an arts and crafts show, a street fair, races and games, fireworks, and a different musical group each of the three nights."

When I asked, "Why do they call it Shanty Days?" the explanation was vague. The name seemed to refer back to the type of dwellings lived in by the early day settlers here.

On Highway 54 immediately after getting off the beach, I went past a couple of gas stations and an area of modest residences, one of which had a life-sized statue of the Blessed Virgin Mary in the front yard. Kind of dull compared to what I saw down the road: a home where the front yard contained a huge statue of the BVM, statues of a Dutch boy and girl, three foxes chasing two geese and beyond that two Dalmatians.

Passing Algoma Motors I stopped, out of curiosity, to compare the cost of a Buick here with the California price and found the prices to be about the same. Some surprise here because, with shipping et al., I had expected the California price to be higher.

From our drive and scouting to Algoma I was already aware of the running conditions today – two-lane road, moderate traffic, fog line to the very edge of the road, seven-foot gravel shoulder, no sightless curves, no steep hills. Piece of cake, especially if I confined myself to the gravel and took no chances with cars. Getting out onto the roadway would be indecent exposure!

Once underway I thought back to how difficult it was to get underway today. Actually I should have been eager– in just two days of running, we would achieve our goal of running across all the lower 48 states.

Today was typical of the many days when I have to coax and cajole myself out of the door to run. What, you thought I'm always bright-eyed and bushy-tailed just squirming to get out the door and run! Not so.

But conversely, never in the 34 years that I've been running, that I've pushed myself out the door, have I ever regretted that I went out. Simply put, I know that I am better for having run.

So thinking, I asked myself, Just how many times in the past 34 years have I gone out to run? That question resulted in some calculating as I went down the road.

No pen and paper in hand I attacked the question like this: 34 years, 365 days a year. Say I ran 345 of those 365 days.

For 10 years that's 3450 days. For 30 years, three times that – and I had to concentrate as I visualized the numbers – 10,350 days.

Now I gotta add four years – 345 times four, 1380 days. So (more concentration and visualization here) the 1380 added to the 10,350 equals 11,730 days.

Okay, now that I have a number, I'd estimate that close to 5000 of those days I had to literally push myself out of the house. Not that I don't like running. But rather than I had to put aside the temptations of watching TV, reading, going shopping, doing a chore or simply yielding to that old demon inertia.

Pretty much the same routine unfolded today on the road – some sights, some observations, some people experiences and the usual heavy dosage of thinking/reflecting/ reminiscing.

Not one spectacular sight all day. What I saw along the way included:

- On the west edges of Algoma I stopped for the simple pleasure of admiring a majestic elm tree in a cemetery and in the process decided that the groundskeeper here deserved an "A" on his report card.
- Cultivated fields, mostly corn and soy beans, and towering grain elevators in every direction.
- St. Johns Lutheran Church, an imposing structure in the boondocks. A Lutheran church with its heavy German affiliation made sense here since more than 50 percent of the state's residents are of German descent, which also makes understandable why nine of Wisconsin's 13 delegates to Congress (two Senators, 11 Congressmen) voted against U.S. entry into World War I.
- As in the past four states crossed, we saw all sorts of uniquely designed mail boxes. Here the predominant themes were a barn, a tractor, a truck, a dairy cow–appropriate for America's dairyland.
- The different barn designs along the way were intriguing. The basic design was similar, in most cases, in that the first story had stone walls and atop it was a second story of frame design with windows that appeared to be living quarters. These U-shaped barns were remindful of similar ones in Europe.
- With all the dairy cows (the state has more than 1.5 million)

the sight of a flock of 100 sheep was unexpected.

- Seeing the Country Bible Church left me wondering, Is there by way of connotation a City Bible Church?

- Off on a small hill 70 yards from the road two guys were setting up a teepee. I watched them arranging the support poles, which didn't seem too intricate if you knew the process. Next chance I get, I'll have to look inside a teepee and see how those poles are arranged. Who knows, if you believe in reincarnation, while I'm doing so there may be an awakening; maybe I'll remember back to being an Indian. One thing I knew for sure about Indians was that if I'd been as good a military tactician as Joseph, Chochise or Geronimo, such knowledge would have enhanced my military career.

- After reading that 352,520 deer were killed in Wisconsin in 1991, I did not expect to see any. On that score I was right. But reading that the state has 15,000 lakes of more than 50 acres, I did expect to see at least one. On that score I was wrong.

Today's sights also included two small towns, Casco and Luxemburg. Casco, a village of 544 souls, provided a brief change of pace in the scenery.

As could be expected, the local bank was the most imposing-looking building in town. The other businesses I saw were a small grocery, a real estate office, a senior home, Jim's Bar and the Red Owl Bar. Small as the town was, it had sidewalks extending three-quarters of a mile, and residences lined both sides of the street.

The residences in Luxemburg, population 1151, were upscale compared to those in Casco. Most of them were constructed of the tawny-colored brick seen so often in these parts.

All the homes had nice lawns but no fences. Was that by ordinance?

I saw that the mascot name for the Casco/Luxembourg high school teams was Spartans – quite appropriate for anybody who endures the winters hereabouts. Across the street was Perry's Nifty 54 Diner, giving rise to the question: Are the kids allowed to cross this highway to go there for lunch, or do they have a closed campus?

To me the centerpiece of town was Stodal's IG Market because the bakery there sells about the best cinnamon rolls I've ever eaten, so I learned on today's drive to the start. Unfortunately Elaine liked them, too, which meant I couldn't stockpile any since she was likely to consume them. Life on the road can be rough!

A few observations resulted as I went down the road:

- Elaine and I agree we're in allergy land because of all the hay, alfalfa, clover being cultivated in the area.
- One of those days when I looked up at the sky, saw patches of blue but also many smoke-colored clouds and fully expected rain, which never materialized.
- Went by a bar I felt like patronizing, "The 54 Run," since I was running Highway 54. I had in hand neither coin for a drink or camera for a photo.
- Amused by the names of some of the towns: Alaska, Poland, Luxemburg. Couldn't figure how Casco got into the act.

A good deal of the thinking/reflecting/reminiscing I did today revolved around things spiritual because this was Sunday. I observed the Sabbath by dwelling a few moments on religious matters. Today I seemed to be sputtering an array of questions, all without any attempt to seek answers.

I began by reflecting back to last Sunday when I talked about God expecting every person to live by a code of conduct. But just what are the common denominators of a code of conduct that God expects every person to follow?

Why is it that a priest – or anyone in a religious order who's taken Sacramental vows, similar to those in the Sacrament of marriage – can simply decide to quit and walk out, and thereafter still be in good graces with the church, whereas a married person who divorces is cut off from the church?

Why can the Catholic church decide, so far into its history, that Saturday is just as good a day as Sunday to observe the Sabbath?

Why are people born blind, deformed, etc.?

Granted that every person has an immortal soul, then it would follow that an innocent infant who dies would go to heaven. What has that infant done to merit eternal happiness?

Why, if you believe the Bible and church teachings, have some people been privileged to witness miracles? That doesn't seem to make for a level playing field. The natural reaction to witnessing a miracle would be to turn saintly.

For that matter what was so special about Saul/Paul that God appeared to him, says the Bible, and asked , in effect, "Saul, why are you persecuting Me?" A similar question could be asked of thousands, millions in fact, "Why are you ignoring Me?"

This same Saul/Paul reported having a vision of heaven, but in describing it all he said was "The eye has not seen, the ear has not heard." That, despite the fact that he was a good writer, was the best he could do. If Paul really had a vision of heaven, why couldn't he give an accurate description of it?

I know a person once a Catholic who had a brief, faulty marriage and, leaving it, tried to get an annulment. He didn't get to first base, despite filing all the correct papers. Why is it that people with money or influence, Kennedys are a good example, can get the Catholic church to annul a marriage?

How can the Catholic church espouse a doctrine that eating meat on a forbidden Friday is a mortal sin that can get a person condemned to hell for eternity?

Why is it that Catholic priests, in the plurality, despite their many years of formal education, are masters at delivering dull, trite sermons that are devoid of any inspirational messages?

What makes me so questioning at this stage in my life, whereas in my younger days I accepted everything on blind faith?

Why is it that whenever I go to church, I notice that at least 75 percent of the congregation consists of old folks? Is it because they are beginning to hear the footsteps of the grim reaper, and they are thus more interested in what will happen on the other side of the fence? A little remindful of the classic movie scene when Edward G. Robinson, a ruthless gangster all his life, has been shot, lies dying and his dying words are a recitation of the Hail Mary.

How does the church explain many passages from the Bible or gospels? Consider just one: "The wife should be subservient to the husband. The husband is the head of the wife. The wife should submit to the husband in all things."

How does the church defend that in today's world? All I could think of, boy, if that were true, what a rallying call for lesbians!

Why is it that there is no room for silence in the Catholic mass today? The place rings with noise – congregation praying, priest chanting or praying, congregation singing. That's not the way it was in my youth.

Has the church decided that people are so addicted to noise that they can't deal with silence? Silence and the thinking it ignites has always been one of the shining attractions of being on the road.

I wondered what a priest hearing all these questions would say. My guess would be, "You need a good weekend retreat to straighten yourself out."

My reaction would probably be, "Padre, it would take a lot longer than a week." I made a mental note to re-read *Razor's Edge*, which I remembered, and I hoped correctly, as the story of a man seeking the true religion.

The day brought two experiences with people. The first happened when I saw a farmer on a tractor approaching me and occupying all the bike lane and much of the gravel shoulder.

I moved another five feet out onto the dirt to get out of his way. He passed without any acknowledgment. If this was an index of Wisconsin, score a minus one.

The second experience occurred when I saw a farmer driving out from his home about 50 yards off the road. Pulling up beside me, he asked, "Are you in trouble?"

"No," I replied. "I'm fine, thanks."

"Are you with that motorhome?" he asked, pointing to Elaine parked 500 yards ahead.

"Yes, that's my pit crew," I told him.

"Okay," he said, then turned around to return to his home.

Nice feeling to know that there are some people who care. This guy had gone to all the trouble to come out and check that I was okay. Score a plus for Wisconsin.

Everything's coming up roses was my feeling when we finished our 16.0-mile day. Our RV park was pleasant, the running was comfortable, the weather was kind, and I was feeling no aches or pains – not even tired.

But I wasn't living it up as much as Elaine, as witnessed by what happened on one occasion when I came into the motorhome and saw her munching on a pastry.

"What is that thing?" I asked.

"It's called a Bismarck," she said. "It's a soft crust filled with whipped cream, and there's chocolate frosting all over the crust. It can't possibly be fattening because it's so light!"

Looking at that thing, nutritionist Covert Bailey would flip out gastronomically. Even I, a bakery junkie, regarded it as overkill.

But, keenly aware that a runner must not ruffle his pit crew, I commented ever so discreetly, "Well, I hope you're enjoying your Bismarck."

She really didn't have to reply, "I just can't tell you how much!"

DAY TWO. I'd gone less than a half-mile this morning when, on the front lawn of a farm house, I saw a jeep with a "For Sale" sign on it. Instantly I had a flashback to an incident that happened to a Marine Corps friend of mine.

In Hawaii during World War II when this friend was a Marine captain, word had reached the Army Headquarters that Marines were stealing Army gear and equipment prior to embarking for combat. Which was a fact.

This incident began when a sergeant in my friend's battalion, loose on liberty, spotted an unmanned Army jeep and decided to commandeer it. He drove it to the ship on which the Marines were embarked and, with the blessings of the battalion CO, the jeep was stowed in the hull of the ship – a welcome gift to the Marines' limited transportation pool.

About the same time that this happened, an Army general appealed to an admiral and requested that all ships with Marines embarked be searched for Army equipment prior to departure. The admiral approved, which meant that the ship with the stolen jeep would be searched.

Hearing this news, the battalion CO paled. He was a regular (not reserve) officer, almost a shoo-in for promotion in wartime. But to be found with that Army jeep would be the kiss of death.

Frantic, he called the captain, my friend, and asked, "What are we going to do?"

"Give me a few minutes," replied the captain, a very bright young officer, "and I'll come up with something, sir."

The plan he devised was to bury the jeep with boxes of K rations Looking into the hold of the ship, a person would think the lower portion was filled entirely with K rations. Or at least that is what the CO hoped, as did the captain who knew he'd be in deep trouble if the jeep were discovered.

When the Army inspection party came aboard, the battalion CO had the duty to accompany it. The captain was told to tag along.

"I've never seen a man so pale – actually white – as the colonel when we came to the jeep area," the captain told me. "When one of the Army guys picked up a carton of K rations and said, 'Damn, you guys must be heavy eaters,' the colonel was actually gasping and half staggered.

"He was sheet white and, thinking he might fall, I got close to be able to catch him. Casually as I could, and trying to come to the colonel's rescue and save my own neck, I quipped, "Well, you know what Napoleon said, 'An army travels on its stomach.' Only in this case it's the Marines."

The captain went on, "Then as the Army inspectors moved on to another area, never did I receive a more grateful look from the colonel than the one he gave me at that moment. And it didn't end there – after the Army folks left, the colonel called me to his stateroom to share some Jack Daniels.

"Later after we landed, we enjoyed the hell out of that jeep. Every time the colonel and I were around it, we exchanged grins."

Now into our fifth day in the Green Bay area Elaine and I were growing fond of the place. We agreed it would be a delightful place to live if it were not so unmercifully cold in winter. Then again, I wasn't too sure I'd want to live in a place that bills itself as the "toilet paper capital of the world."

Being in the area so long, we learned these tidbits about Green Bay: that, settled in 1764, it's the oldest community in Wisconsin; that, some surprise here, the world's first automobile race, 1878, started in Green Bay and the steam-powered cars raced to Madison; that the Green Bay Packers were once known as the Indians (because they were sponsored by the Indian Packing Company).

In all our 48 state crossings, we'd never stayed in one city so long. Enjoying ourselves, we would have been reluctant to leave except that after today we would be heading home after a 2-1/2-month absence.

The setting today was a replica of yesterday, road conditions being exactly the same, and dairy farms, barns and silos always being within sight. A unique feature of some of the dairy farms, so we learned, is that they offer family vacations (days or weekends) with lodging and meals for people interested in observing and learning the dairy operation. By now I'd gone by enough dairy farms and their lung-engulfing odors (not talking roses here!) to find such a vacation unappealing.

I had to admire the Wisconsin dairymen for their restraint. The state leads the nation in cheese production (colby and brick cheese were developed here), yet across the entire peninsula I saw only one sign reading "Cheese for sale." Contrast that with Vermont where just about every mile we saw a "Maple syrup for sale" sign.

About midway through this day it hit me that this would be the last day Elaine, pit crewing, and I, running, would be doing our thing across a state.

True, after Wisconsin we had two states left, Alaska and Hawaii. But on those runs we'd fly to the state, then rent a car for the run.

Today was the end of the line for the motorhome as far as our state runs were concerned. Of course, we were still dependent on it for the long trip home.

At one point today some small birds, evidently judging me too close to their nests, started dive bombing me. Their antics resurrected memories of Wyoming where this was a frequent occurrence.

Today's sights also included three homes with large statues of the Blessed Virgin Mary, unusual to me inasmuch as I did not see one such statue in my 3192-mile run across the USA. Something new and different for Wisconsin when a llama family – father, mother, child– ambled to a fence to get a closer look at me.

The closest I came to being in any town today was passing through the New Franken area where I saw only residences. A sign pointed to the town itself, one mile away.

Thanks but no thanks. It would take something drastic for me to go a mile out of my way. Something drastic like a promise that, arriving there, I'd witness Clinton signing his resignation papers – plenty of incentive there!

Today's people experiences revolved around a farmer, a kid, two women and an old gent. The farmer experience was similar to yesterday.

When he approached me driving his tractor and taking all the bike lane and some of the road, I decided to cross the road and give him more space. I was curious to see if he'd acknowledge me by waving a thanks, and he didn't. Like I said, similar to yesterday.

The kid, I guessed him to be about eight, was driving a four-wheel go-cart on a farm road. Looked like fun, but my concern was, would this kid be mobile all his life, always depending on wheels, never exercising? The odds were that would be his lifestyle.

Two women, walking, approached, and I greeted them with "Hi." They returned the greeting.

But when I asked, "How cold does it get here in the winter?" their body language spoke, "Get lost, old man." Probably thought I was some sort of kook–a bit understandable considering how often they see an 80-year-old in T-shirt, shorts and beat-up shoes, plodding down this road.

The old gent, out on the road to pick up his mail, appeared friendly enough. After we exchanged greetings, I asked, "Can you answer a question that's been on my mind – why do they call Wisconsin the Badger State?"

"Oh, that's easy," he said. "It comes from the early miners in the southwest part of the state who were called 'badgers' because they burrowed into the hills."

Mulling that as I went down the road, I thought about California gold miners and their panning. It was a wonder that someone did not think of calling them 'dead pans'!

One passing thought today was that I felt like a damn sissy doing this easy run when I compared myself with a couple of guys who braved it. One was Terry Fox, cancer victim and amputee, who ran across most of Canada. When Elaine and I were in Ottawa, I stood beside his bronze statue and Elaine photographed me, proud to be in such company.

A million or more people have heard about Terry. But I'd bet not a thousand have heard of Charles F. Lummis, a 25-year-old journalist, who in 1884 left Ohio for a 3507-mile walk to the West Coast.

On the road 143 days he crossed eight states and territories, often going hungry and escaping from danger He made the journey because he "wanted to experience a long pedestrian tour" and because he "felt ashamed to know so little about America."

He told his story in a book titled *A Tramp Across the Continent*. Reading it, I felt like a prima donna doing what I was doing.

On a lighter note I recalled the ingenuity of a friend of mine when I was an administrator in the Sacramento City Schools. He submitted a requisition for a TV for his department, but the purchasing department turned him down.

He waited two weeks, then submitted another requisition, this one included a long list of electronic parts. This one the purchasing department approved, not realizing that all those parts added up to all the components of a TV set.

My friend enjoyed his TV, and the purchasing department never knew. Little wonder that this guy went on to become a superintendent!

Sort of found myself thinking at times today about some of my friends, dead and alive:

• Dan Halvorsen, dead in his 50s from a brain cancer. Especially remembered running the Boston Marathon with him because he ran interference for me in the crowded field of runners.

• Dick Houston, also dead in his 50s from colon cancer. Three things about Dick popped out – that even after he had a colostomy, he took on running the tough Crater Lake Marathon; that, knowing he was dying and although he was suffering, he came to a race for the express purpose – unspoken – to say goodbye to friends; that, so I learned only at his memorial, he was an experienced mountain climber (one of those brave souls whose lives depend on ropes and pitons).

I also thought back to the 80th birthday party Elaine insisted on giving me last April and the humorous remarks that Pete League, Jeremiah Russel, Abe Underwood, Jay Kenagy and Jon Brown made about me. An old grunt Marine should not admit this (damages the image!), but I got misty-eyed remembering that a couple of them said, "We love you, man!"

The runners there that night must have done a good job because after hearing them Dr. Al Sessarego, a retired superintendent and my former boss, said he regretted not belonging to the running fraternity. Of the many bosses I've worked for in my two careers, none was better than Al.

And his was the best of many job interviews. It consisted of these words: "Do you want the job or not?"

Thinking of Al, an educator, conjured up what I consider one of the biggest inequalities of education: It fails to adequately reward competence and to penalize incompetence.

As but one example, teachers and coaches who devote inordinate hours, much effort and work, and considerable talent to their jobs – coaches like Al Baeta, Walt Lange, Mil Frederick immediately come to mind – are not properly recognized and rewarded (except for the satisfaction they get from helping people). At the same time incompetents, much to the detriment of students, are carried until retirement.

I could cite a litany of names here, but that would be to no avail. The worst case I saw here was an incompetent teacher who had been dismissed returned to the classroom by judicial ruling. Once back in the classroom, he continued his "teaching," which consisted of having the students copy names and addresses from the phone book.

Then my thinking swung back again to my friend Jeremiah Russell He had chided me for mentioning roadkill in *Ten Million Steps*. One of the first things I plan to do when returning home is to call Jeremiah and tell him that the job of the Wisconsin Volunteers for the Home Habitat Society is to count roadkill along the roadsides.

Back to the moment and the road when I realized that for a long spell I have not reported on running shoes, a subject dear to runners' hearts. For the record, across every state this year I've worn the same brand and model of 8.5-ounce racing flats. Not training shoes, not heavily cushioned shoes but racing flats – same brand, same model, four different pairs.

Like the great Jack Foster, I believe in wearing the lightest shoe I can get away with (i.e., avoid injury) while wearing it. The current shoes are the most protective racing flats I've ever worn, good even on the gravel.

I never wear socks with running shoes and, sockless throughout this trip, I got not a single blister. I don't want to give an endorsement for the company and brand, which is a reciprocal agreement since the company would never consider paying me for an endorsement.

Once I crossed Highway 57, the north-south road on the west side of the peninsula, I knew I was nearing the finish. Running on Highway 1 and on top of a knoll, I could see the water ahead and realized that when I reached it; I would complete running across all the lower 48 states.

But I didn't feel the high, the glow I felt upon finishing the USA run. Maybe the excitement was dimmed from the fact that the running across states was becoming old hat. Also it was spread over such a long period, six summers versus the 124 consecutive days of the USA run.

While on Algoma Road I did get a look at the adjacent campus of University of Wisconsin/Green Bay. It appeared quite attractive but, at least to my knowledge, it could not boost of a neon graduate like UW/Superior that graduated Arnold Schwarzenegger.

Algoma turned into Scottwood Drive, which I followed until it intersected with Nicholet, where I turned east and ran to the finish at Ommuniversit Park and the waters of Green Bay.

After I finished, Elaine took the usual photos of our finishing a state.

"You know," she said, "when you were finishing, I wanted to yell to all the people in the park that you were finishing running across all the lower 48 states. I think this is a bigger achievement than the run across the country."

I thought about that a moment. "Well, I guess it is," I said. "A lot of people have run across the country, but I don't think anyone else has run across all the lower 48 states.

"And we are talking about 7593 miles of running, jogging, walking without counting Alaska and Hawaii. Even though I ran the shortest distances this summer, that's still a lot of miles."

The day over, I reflected on running the 48 states. I'd run in temperatures as low as 10 degrees and as high as 106 degrees, in 100-percent humidity, in pelting rain and storms, even in snow one day, and as low as sea level and as high as Monarch Pass at 11,312 feet.

I'd seen God's handiwork while running, beautiful deserts, majestic mountains, cascading streams, glorious sunrises. I'd crossed many of America's major rivers – the Mississippi, the Ohio, the Missouri, the Delaware, among others.

I'd enjoyed food and drink from the more than 2500 pit stops Elaine made while often finding parking a problem. And all along the way I enjoyed her companionship and encouragement. Tasting a small part of each of the 48 states, Elaine and I were awed and humbled by the vastness and the resources of our country.

Above all we were grateful to God that we were blessed to enjoy the experience and that both of us survived it with no injuries or illnesses. Considering that we were on the road 550 days in the motorhome while crossing 48 states, that's beating the odds.

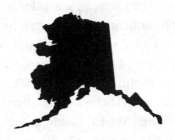

Chapter 22

Alaska

Klondike Highway 2 and White Pass

Date: *August 15th, 1997*
Miles: *15.5*
Route: *Start on Klondike Highway, Highway 2, at British Columbia and north Alaska border and follow Klondike Highway south to Skagway and water, south border of Alaska.*

Bears, unkind weather and a narrow, curvy, mountainous road – those were my apprehensions as I thought about running Alaska. Timber wolves would have appeared on that listing had I been aware of their ferocity and 240-pound size.

But not to worry – as Alaska unfolded, none of these apprehensions materialized. In fact, just about everything about Alaska came up smelling of roses.

This good luck started when we checked in for our flight from Sacramento to Juneau and discovered we could upgrade to first class for $160 for the two of us. We did, and doing so entered a world of travel we'd never experienced before – comfortable leather seats, relaxing leg and arm room , food served with china and silverware (versus plastic and paper).

The first-class experience shares some commonality with experiencing drugs – it's exhilarating, expensive and addicting. Let me hastily add that I've never done drugs, so on that score I'm dealing with hearsay. I've done a lot of economy travel, though, and returning to it after tasting the luxury of first-class will be punishing.

En route from Seattle to Juneau the pilot announced that he was battling 160-mile-per-hour headwinds. From where we sat in first-class, we would never have know without his informing us. I wondered if the passengers in the back of the plane were similarly unaffected.

At Juneau for our flight to Skagway – 85 miles and 45 minutes away – we skidded from first-class to a three-passenger propelled Cessna operated by Wings Alaska. Elaine occupied the co-pilot's seat and, seated behind her, I was the only other passenger.

After Elaine told Brian, the young pilot (his uniform was ball cap, plaid shirt, Levi's and Adidas running shoes) that she hoped so see some bears, he hugged the mountains trying to locate one for her. All I could think of was, What is the word for that force that emanates from mountains and causes planes to crash? Whatever the word, I hoped that none of it was about today. White-knuckle stuff here.

As we approached the postage-stamp airport at Skagway, the pilot cautioned, "Now don't get nervous when I fly into the pass and make a tight right turn. I've got to do that to land into the wind."

As he executed the maneuver, making the U-turn left to right, the plane first played tag with the mountains on the left and after that with the mountains on the right. Lucky he had warned us. Otherwise I would have been properly attired if wearing a pair of Depends.

The Alaska running route I planned would take us from a bit north of the British Columbia border, south down Klondike Highway 2 (Highway 98) through White Pass to the water's edge at Skagway – a mere 15.4 miles.

All I knew about the route was what I had garnered from reading *Milepost* (one of the best travel guides to Alaska) and from corresponding with David Sexton, the police chief of Skagway, and Roy Reisinger, a runner who lives in Alaska.

Milepost told me, "Klondike Highway 2 is a two-lane asphalt-surfaced road... There is a steep 11.5-mile/18.5-kilometer grade between Skagway and White Pass that is narrow and winding."

Milepost provided a Cook's Tour on what I'd see along the route. To cite just a few tidbits of detailed description, I was told that, counting from the British Columbia/Alaska border southward, I'd see these sights at mileages indicated:

0.5 mile: White Pass summit, elevation 3290 feet

3.4 miles: Capt. William Moore Bridge, Skagway River gorge

5.9 miles: Historical plaque honoring miners of the Klondike Gold Rush

8.9 miles: U.S. Customs station

12.0 miles: End of downhill descent that began at White Horse Pass summit

12.7 miles: Dyea road junction

13.4 miles: Skagway River Bridge.

Chief Sexton had written, "You should encounter no wildlife problems. RV's, tour buses and ore trucks are a much greater risk."

The chief also asked, "Are you aware of the Klondike Road Relay (more than 1000 runners) Sept. 12 and 13?" That I was aware of because I had read about it in Don Kardong's book, *Hills, Hawgs, and Ho Chi Minh* – which among other things Roy Reisinger had mentioned in his correspondence.

On the day after we arrived in Skagway, as Elaine climbed behind the wheel of our rented Camry to drive to the British Columbia border, I was bubbling with curiosity over what I'd see along the way by way of wildlife, road conditions and vehicular traffic. I had full expectations of seeing a narrow, twisty, two-lane road.

I blossomed when I saw a road with wide lanes, gentle curves and even a small bike lane. As we continued the drive uphill, I kept thinking, It'll get narrow and curvy soon.

While I was jumping with joy over this road being considerably better running than I had expected, Elaine was dripping with disappointment. She wanted to see bears and (how lucky can I get!) none were about.

The drive verified what *Milepost* had said about the route. The first half-mile would be uphill, followed by a steep descent of 11.5 miles, and after that a flat surface to the water's edge.

The road was kind; the traffic light enough to be manageable. My only remaining concern: Was any wildlife lurking roadside?

Ever the brave one, I decided to carry my .45 Colt pistol in my fanny pack, even though it weighed more than four pounds. Doing so, I realized this was mainly for emotional relief (go down fighting!) as opposed to being a safety factor because I'd seen the size of Alaska bears and realized that a .45 would antagonize (rather than stop) one.

I wound up carrying the .45 for only half the run because, a mile before arriving at the U.S. Customs station, I took it from my fanny pack and hid it in the trunk of the Camry.

I started the run a bit behind (north of) the border on a semi-flat stretch of road to warm up for the upcoming climb of a half-mile. Once I hit the downhill, I ran continuously for the 11.5 miles until I reached the flat surface, stopping only for Elaine's two-mile pit stops visits and refueling.

At each pit stop Elaine reported she was busily scanning the hills with her binoculars and had seen no wildlife. On the positive side she was very taken with the performance of the Camry – almost to the point where I thought she might announce she was trading her car for a Camry.

At one pit stop Elaine discovered only after I'd arrived that she was parked beside a berry patch, but one not frequented at the moment by bears – at least not one that we could see.

(I should parenthetically inject here that the day after we finished our run, I talked with a ranger who had just driven over our route, and he told me that he had to wait behind a long line of cars whose drivers were gawking at a couple of bears munching on the grass in a meadow area near the road.)

While waiting at pit stops, Elaine was annoyed by mosquitoes, humorously called "flying hypodermic syringes" and "Alaska's state bird." While running I had no mosquito problems, but they did descend on me at pit stops.

The scenery during the entire route was awesome. Some mountains majestic and snow-capped; some mountains rocky and intimidating, inhospitable; others hosts to heavy forestation.

The fast flowing Skagway River, in the canyon to my left was in sight and sound much of the way. I wandered in a world of wonderment.

Because *Milepost* had given me so many landmarks and mileages along the way, I was aware at all times of exactly where I was – how far I'd gone, how far I had to go. It doesn't get much easier.

From the point where I started the run downhill, the running was like times past as I went along almost effortlessly. I was encouraged and elated with how easy it was.

Even Elaine took notice, saying, "You're running just like you did when you were fast. I was really surprised to see you coming down the hill so fast."

My asthma must have been on vacation because I had no breathing problems. Another problem I had worried about before starting was an abdominal pain I'd been experiencing the past couple of months. I had feared that all the downhill running would strain it and that, as a result, I'd be hurting or temporarily halted by pain.

One MD had diagnosed the pain as muscular-skeletal – if that were true, it seemed to me that the downhill would aggravate it. Surprisingly not once during the entire 15.4-mile effort did I feel any abdominal discomfort, a fact that I did not realize until after I'd finished the run because doing it I was too occupied with my surroundings, the threat of bears and road traffic to even think about the problem.

At water's edge when I was finishing, Elaine said, "We should have some fanfare here. A big celebration you've now finished all 50 states. The only person to ever do so."

"Well, 49-3/4 states to be technical," I reminded her. "I still have nine miles of Hawaii to do before finishing the 50th state."

"Not in my book," she replied. "You already ran across Hawaii. You and Paff just want that silly business of getting down to the ocean."

By getting down to the ocean, she was referring to the plan that Dr. Ralph Paffenbarger and I have to go from the town of Honokaa to Waipio Valley and the ocean beach there.

"Ah," I retorted, "but think of the dramatic value of it – the 50th state as the 50th state run."

Her reply: "Dumb, dumb, dumb."

That reference was to her contention that Paff and I had already completed Hawaii back in March, when we'd crossed from the west side to the east side on Highway 19, ending just a bit to the east of Honokaa.

One sign for me of a good run is that I am hungry afterwards. And so it was with Alaska. On the route through Skagway I'd spotted the 21 Siding Restaurant, which looked inviting.

I suggested to Elaine that we have a celebration lunch there. What we both ordered would cause Covert Bailey to shake his head in dismay. Nonetheless we enjoyed our avocado, cheddar and crabmeat sandwiches on sourdough bread.

Over lunch Elaine and I reviewed the Alaska run and decided that it was the best of the 22 states we crossed this year. For scenery no other state even came close. Running conditions, road and traffic, were better than most of the other 21 states.

Even with weather we lucked out – a warm, clear, bright day. And we came away from the experience learning a bit about historic White Pass where men and horses struggled and died on their way to the Klondike Gold Rush.

Knowing that Elaine was still focused on wanting to see a bear, and having time and a rented car on our hands, I suggested that we drive to the deserted town of Dyea, 10 miles–eight of which are dirt road– in the hope of seeing wildlife. Drive we did, see wildlife we did not. (If I were a real chivalrous soul, I could satisfy her bear urge by taking her to Admiralty Island, which is home to more than 1600 brown bears – at least one per square mile.)

But the trip did give us a look into history since the park service displays there provided information about Dyea which flourished in the gold rush days. These days Dyea is the trailhead for the Chilkoot Trail, a strenuous but popular 33-mile hike. I made a mental note to send my friend Mike Tymn info about this trail since he has a yen to try some wilderness hiking.

Come to think of it, I should also tell my Marine classmate Andy Bissett. He and his wife Holly like to hike wilderness trails. Unlike me they embrace seeing bears.

Not seeing any wildlife around Dyea, nor any on our run, Elaine decided to focus on something at which she excels. The result: a spending spree in Skagway, vigorously exercising her Visa card as we shopped in every store in town.

Unfortunately I got sucked into this spending frenzy. A by-product of this was a couple of pregnant suitcases on our trip home.

These days the main drag of Skagway is about five blocks long with shops, restaurants and a couple of hotels lining both sides of the street. Tourists flocking ashore from cruise ships, docked three blocks from downtown, bolster the economy.

The tourist season extends from mid-May to mid-September. The year-around population varies from 600 to 800, depending on the source of this information. Back in the Klondike Gold Rush days the population zoomed to 20,000 as boatloads of stampeders landed here.

Our original plan for Alaska called for us to fly to Juneau, then take the ferry to Skagway. Unable to make the ferry travel arrangements, we scheduled flights between Juneau and Skagway.

After we arrived in Skagway, we checked into ferry travel and found that, indeed, we could get ticketed from Skagway to Juneau and also get an outside stateroom.

The seven-hour trip through the Inside Passage, with all its spectacular scenery, was delightful. The Alaska state ferry system considerably exceeded expectations.

The fare for the two of us was $52. The outside cabin, costing $34, included two bunk beds (guess who got the top one!), a sink, shower and commode.

The ship's cafeteria menu included a wide selection at reasonable prices. Borderline luxury at bargain-basement prices (as proof of that, consider that an Amtrak roomette – consisting of only two bunks, no sink, no commode – costs $135 for the 130-mile trip from Sacramento, California, to Reno, Nevada). The only downside to the ferry experience was having to be at the terminal by 5:30 A.M.

On the ferry trip to Juneau Elaine told me that the highlight of the trip for her was sitting in the co-pilot's seat on the flight from Juneau to Skagway, searching the hills for bears and enjoying the scenery.

"What did you enjoy most?" she asked me.

"Two things," I replied. "The relief felt on the drive to the start when I saw how kind the road was. And second, the discovery on starting that I was primed for running downhill."

Then, waxing diplomatic, I added, "Of course, both of those are secondary to the great company and pit crewing."

"It won't work," she answered. "No way am I going to Hawaii."

She was referring to her previously announced decision not to travel to Hawaii with Paff and me and to pit crew there for us. "I've already told you it's too hot for me to enjoy, and besides, as I said before, that nine-mile thing is dumb."

I had hoped that the Alaska adventure might persuade her to change her mind about Hawaii. I now realized that my chances of that were on par with winning the Lotto.

No cause for tears here, though – let's face it, I have been blessed with her companionship and pit crewing that carried me through 49-3/4 states. The single most memorable and meaningful treasure that I take away from all those states is our sharing – of both the good and the bad.

I'll miss her as I trudge all those "dumb" nine miles in Hawaii.

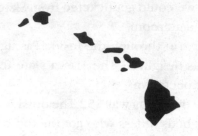

Chapter 23

Hawaii

An Odyssey Ends Here

Date: *February 27th and 28th, March 1st, December 11th, 1997*
Miles: *37.8*
Route: *Start at Pacific on west side of Hawaii at Spencer Beach County Park, exit park, follow Highway 270 south to its junction with Highway 19. Follow 19 east to Honokaa, and there take 270 north to Waipio Overlook. Follow marked road to Waipio State Park Beach and Pacific Ocean, east border of Hawaii.*

Just as Alaska was the 49th state admitted to the Union and our 49th state run, I connived (I'll explain this later) that Hawaii, 50th state admitted, would be our 50th state to run. From the outset of my Hawaii planning, the island that I planned to run across, was the island of Hawaii itself.

Since it was such a short distance across, I could afford to take on the biggest island in the Hawaiian chain – especially since I would run only one island. No way was I about to take on more than one. After all, Hawaii's chain of 132 reefs, shoals and islands extends 1600 miles across the Pacific Ocean.

Time was, though, when I would have liked to run more than one island. This was back in the days when there was an organized race, called the Great Hawaiian Footrace in which the competitors spent a week or so on racing routes in several different islands. Much as I would have liked to participate, the entry fee of $1200 deterred me.

Another part of my planning was that since Hawaii would mark the completion of our 50-state odyssey, I hoped to make it fun – maybe even somewhat festive. Those considerations in mind, and wanting to savor the excitement of reaching our goal of 50 states (becoming the only person ever to do so), I got the idea that having a friend make the pilgrimage with me would add to my enjoyment.

With that thought, the name Ralph Paffenbarger flashed into my mind. Paff and I have run 1200 miles alongside each other in races – including such famous ones as the Comrades (90-kilometer) Marathon in South Africa, the London Marathon and about 10 Honolulu Marathons. I was his pit-crew captain when at age 61 he set a 60-plus record of 22 hours, three minutes for the Western States 100-Mile Endurance Run – a punishing grind up and down the Sierra Nevada, a race in which the runners gain about 20,000 feet in elevation and lose about the same number. Normally a genteel and gentlemanly sort and a scholar extraordinare, Paff exploded with animal ferocity whenever unleashed on the Western States Trail. He finished that grueling race five times, and was one of only three finishers in the very first WST race.

But that was then – good Lord, all the way back to 1984, prior to his heart attack and subsequent operation. And this is now – now when Paff is limited to walking and, I suspect, grateful to be alive and able to be capable of that.

Now being so, I knew that if I asked Paff about accompanying me across Hawaii it would mean we'd be limited to a brisk walk, not a run. Reflecting on that, I thought, So what?

My goal has always been just to get across a state, enjoy the experience, speed being of little consideration. Besides, walking would give me more time to savor the Hawaii experience, and I'd be doing it in good company.

I had little doubt when I wrote to Paff to ask him if he'd like to indulge in one Last Hurrah by going across Hawaii with me that he'd accept, adventurous soul that he is. Inviting him, and after conferring with Elaine, I laid down three rules: We walk, we limit each day to nine miles, and he hoists a red flag if he gets weary or woozy. We based the nine miles, a big jump from his daily average of three miles, on getting across the island in three days. I made him clearly understand that if he had to rely on me for CPR, he could consider himself dead.

The very day my invitation arrived at Paff's home, he called and enthusiastically enlisted in the Hawaii venture. His acceptance was about as expected as listening to Rush Limbaugh and expecting to hear his bragging and ego inflation.

Our battle plan called for Elaine to drive a rental car and to pit crew for us. She and I had two secret covenants of our own:

1. The pit stops would be every two miles, instead of the usual three.
2. We would both monitor Paff because we were both aware of his fierce competitive spirit and resolute will power, and we feared he might go into denial if he got into trouble. We decided that either of us could declare "cease fire" if one of us detected Paff bordering on trouble.

Thus with Paff, Elaine and me – two runners (er, walkers) and pit crew, roles we'd played in hundreds of miles in races – the cast was set for the final chapter in our drama of 50-state crossings.

DAY ONE. At the sea, precisely at Spencer Beach County Park on the western side of Hawaii, Elaine posed Paff and me for a photo before we started the trek across the island. We lined up with the Spencer Beach County Park sign as a backdrop, and I was sure the sign would come out looking better in the photo than us, for such are the perils of age.

The photo session over, I told Paff, "Okay, now the rules call for us to touch our feet in the water on this western side before starting across to the eastern side."

Obliging soul that he is, Paff did not ask, "What rules?" Instead he said, "Let's do it," and we headed for the water where we gingerly dipped the toes of our shoes. No need to be macho here and douse our expensive shoes in salt water!

Our next chore was to work our way uphill 600 yards or so out of the park and onto Highway 270. As we did so, a light rain began to fall and it continued for our first four miles. Actually it was warm and semi-refreshing.

Following 270 south for half a mile we came to Highway 19 east which would be our route across the island. I was fully confident that 19 was runnable because my daughter Nancy and her husband, Dan Phillips, had scouted it for me while on a trip to Hawaii a couple of months ago.

Runnable meant the road had a couple of feet or so of shoulder on each side to which Paff and I could retreat when cars approached. Luckily for us the two-lane road was lightly traveled, and most of the drivers were considerate enough to move over for us.

The first four miles were sparsely populated, just a small scattering of homes. The first eye-catcher, this at 4.5 miles, was the Hawaiian Fresh Egg Ranch with 10 chicken sheds, each 50 yards long by my estimate. By now I was aware that every step since leaving the water had been uphill.

At both the two- and four-mile pit stops we took time out to drink in the scenery. Not much to see as we looked ahead to the upward road leading toward the Waimea plateau. But looking back to the east, we got some spectacular views of the ocean and the coastline.

A bit to the southeast stood Mauna Kea mountain bedecked with snow. "You know," I told Paff, "I hiked that mountain in 1963. At the time the infantry battalion I commanded – Third Battalion, Fourth Marines – was training for 10 days at Pohakuloa training facility at the base of the mountain, and every day I looked at the mountain and wondered if I could climb it."

"Was it a tough climb?" Paff asked.

"No, not really. In your prime you could have jogged all the way to the top. My biggest problem was avoiding the wild boar that roam the mountain."

"The view from the top must have made the climb worthwhile," Paff said.

"I didn't luck out there because of the clouds near the summit. But I did catch sight of Mauna Loa, the other big mountain on the island, sort of peaking out through the clouds.

"The sight I remember most was the hundreds of boulders – granite, I guess. Later I learned that these rocks were remains of an ancient glacier that once covered the top of the mountain."

"What's the elevation at the top?" Paff asked.

"It's 13,796 feet. You know, after you've hiked one of these things, the elevation sticks with you. Like Pike's Peak being 14,110 feet, Mt. Fuji 12,388 feet and Monarch Pass, which I crossed on the USA run, being 11,312 feet."

"Pike's Peak I remember well from my race, 28 miles up and down that year," Paff replied. Yes, I thought, and even though you're too modest to remind me, I know you won a belt-buckle award because of your superior performance, and you broke the 40-plus record for the ascent.

Gazing at Mauna Kea, I said, "We're pretty lucky to be seeing the beauty of the mountain capped with such a heavy snow. When I hiked it, I was told it snows there only between December and May, and the amount varies from year to year.

"But there seems to be enough snow to keep an outfit called Ski Guides Hawaii in business. They rent skis and even provide a lift to the snow. I also have heard about the Hawaii Ski Association."

"That's news to me," Paff commented. "I'd bet that not even one percent of the Hawaii tourists are aware that skiing is available on the islands."

As we continued up the hill, I was surprised to see Elaine parked almost a mile short of the six-mile pit stop. "Got a problem?" I asked.

"No problem," she replied. "Just a suggestion. This is supposed to be a fun thing, so how about taking a break and driving into Waimea for lunch."

That was an easy sell. Paff and I bought it instantly. In fact, we even allowed Elaine a few minutes of store-browsing – as if we had any other choice!

Back on the road, we'd gone a little over a mile – actually being 6.5 miles into our day – when we noticed a sign giving the elevation at 2000 feet. Darn thing was bilingual because it also gave the height in meters, 610 to be exact.

As we were reading the sign, a lady in a flashy red convertible stopped to ask if we needed a ride. My guess, she was thinking: Two forlorn fossils, fugitives from the Shady Pines Rest Home.

But, hey, wait a minute, I found myself thinking, What gives here? At around eight miles a young lady in a Jeep wrangler stopped to ask if we needed a ride. When on the road alone, I got no ride offers from young and attractive women. Now here I am with Paff getting two such offers.

Does this guy have some compelling charm, some fatal attraction that eludes me? Or could the scenario be that the two of us together are such a pathetic sight that we scream for rescue. Sorry, Paff, but that seems the more likely version.

The biggest cluster of residences we saw all day was at the junction of Highways 19 and 250. A sign indicated that 250 lead to Hawi, 20 miles north.

"Too bad we don't have time to drive that road," I told Paff. "It's supposed to be one of the most picturesque roads on the island."

In another 50 yards, and 8.7 miles into our day, as we came to the Kamuela Museum, I heard Paff say, "We're going to have to take a look at this."

Even though I was not sure we had the time, I could not play Scrooge by saying no. But it turned out that there was no need to say no because the museum, the largest private one in the state, appeared to be closed. Even if it were open, between us we were not carrying the $10 required for our entry fees.

At nine miles, and an elevation of 2,500 feet, we had just about reached the Waimea plateau. We talked Elaine into letting us extend the day to 9.7 miles so we could finish at a distinctive landmark- the historic Hale Kea, a spacious white frame home restored as a visitor attraction. I estimated the building and surrounding grounds to be worth a considerable fortune, a judgment based on just having passed the Sandalwood Housing Development where homes were priced at $495,000 and lots at $170,000.

On our way back to our hotel in Kona, Elaine, Paff and I assessed our day. "I was tired," Paff reported. "but I held up better than expected. I'll be ready for an encore tomorrow."

"Seeing you two talking and carrying on all the time sort of reminded me of old times and many races," Elaine said. "I could tell you were enjoying yourselves even though you're not the tigers you used to be."

She had analyzed it rather well, I thought: Paff and I were having a good time despite the dramatic decline in our athletic ability. The unspoken and undeniable fact was that each of us – he as a heart attack survivor, me as a cancer survivor – was grateful just to be alive, to be active, to be fully functional physically and mentally.

Once again I marveled at how such a simple act – doing this walking with a close friend – could overflow my day with joy. Who needs drugs?

On a lighter note, and answering Elaine, I said, "Well, I'd have to say that your suggested lunch break helped to keep us fueled up. That's a must for tomorrow."

"Which reminds me," Paff said, "where are we going to have dinner?"

Ah yes, this guy was fully okay. Elaine and I didn't have to worry about him being ready for tomorrow.

DAY TWO. On the 40-mile drive to the start of our second day in Hawaii, Paff and I reminisced about the 10 times we ran the Honolulu Marathon. One of our favorite memories revolved around the warmup period before the race.

Here we had discovered gold because we fared so much better than the other runners who lined up to use a portable potty, who warmed up in restricted running space, who might even be caught in rain or a drizzle. Contrastingly Paff and I had discovered an indoor garage where, courtesy of the attendant, we had a private rest room, considerable space to jog and warm up, and shelter from any rain.

Year after year we returned to this refuge, each time surprised and pleased to find it available and exclusively ours. Kind of tough, though, once race time approached to leave this regal setting and become a peasant with the rest of the runners.

Getting underway today, we did not generate quite the excitement of yesterday when Paff was unsure of his condition. Now he was fully confident of handling nine miles or so.

His confidence concerned Elaine and me a bit because he's such a hard man to discourage once launched on a cause or mission. We were afraid he might get grandiose ideas about doing the entire 18 miles to Honokaa. No matter how good he felt, Elaine and I were resolved to end the day around nine miles.

We started on Highway 19 a mile or so to the west of Waimea. By now we reached the 2500-foot elevation of the plain or plateau on which Waimea sits, a plateau extending south all the way to the base of Mauna Kea. The northern edge of Waimea lies at the foot of the Kohala mountains.

And that sorted our setting for the day – the Kohala mountains on our left, the Waimea plateau crowded with businesses and residences dead ahead, and towering Mauna Kea to our right.

Having driven through Waimea a number of times before, we were in familiar territory. If we did not know already, we would not have to be rocket scientists to deduce who owns the town. Just walk through the town, as we did, and see a dozen or so signs with Parker Ranch on them (Parker Ranch Shopping Center, Parker Ranch Lodge, etc.) and you'll know.

From previous trips we were acquainted with Parker Ranch, the largest privately owned ranch in U.S.– 225,000 acres, 50,000 head of cattle and 1000 horses. Hey, pardner, that's a spread to stir up envy in even a Texas cattle baron!

To put it in perspective, those 225,000 acres are about three-fourths the size of Oahu, one hell of a lot of real estate (thinking in terms of money, remember those lots we saw yesterday at Sandalwood cost $170,000, a mere lot). This holding was born when John Palmer Parker, a young seaman about 19 or so, jumped ship in 1809 and wound up at Hawaii, where he married a granddaughter of Kamehameha.

Actually the name Waimea ("red water" in Hawaiian) is almost an affront to the Parker heritage. More to the Parker tradition, the town is also known as Kamuela (Hawaiian for "Samuel") and was named after Parker's grandson, and the official post office address is Kamuela. Most maps show both names (Waimea, Kamuela), but my guess is that 90 percent of the tourists know it only as Waimea.

As Paff and I passed through the town at a walking pace, as apart from a fast drive, I became more aware of how the town was growing, moving in the direction of urbanization instead of revolving entirely around ranching. Motels, restaurants and shopping centers were all about.

In the downtown area we passed a good-sized, modern hospital and across the street from it an observatory. I did note one historic building – the Imiola Church, built in 1857 – which was just a short distance east of the Parker Ranch Shopping Center.

As we walked through the area, it became apparent in much finer detail than on our previous drives that Waimea is split down the middle, east and west – the east being the wet side, the west the dry side. The first half of our day was through the dry side, the second half through lush and green pastures and rolling hills.

All through town Paff and I exchanged comments on the sights and setting. At one point we both came up with the same observation: We had not seen one bookstore among the many stores along the way. A message there maybe.

Ever seeking fortification for our endeavors, Paff took note of a specialty ice cream store and I spotted a bakery. We solemnly vowed to stop at both on our drive back to the hotel. This promise of things to come caused us to move forward with renewed vigor.

Once we edged into the eastern area, we saw a proliferation of

"Home for Sale" signs. This tied-in with what I'd read – housing is very available on the eastside and the prices are considerably less that on the west where houses are hard to come by.

Shortly after we left the built-up area, I heard Paff say, "I've just calculated that I'm five years, six months, four days younger than you."

The guy's brain is never out of gear, I thought. "Well," I replied, "in this twosome that makes me the guru."

Without a moment's hesitation Paff said, "Not too sure about that. My impression is a guru has to be venerable. Need I say more?"

He knew me too well for me to even attempt to answer. As for knowing him, I recalled some of the things I knew: that he started thinking about becoming an MD as early as the fifth grade when he was diagnosed with mastoiditis, had an operation, and spent 11 days in a hospital; that he graduated from Ohio State University (where his father was a professor) and that he attended Northwestern Medical School; that among the 5000 or so epidemiologists in the country, he is one of the most highly respected; that he has won a number of distinguished professional awards, the most recent being the 1996 International Olympic Committee's Olympic prize for Sports Science; that socially the guy is probably the most gracious person I know; that as a friend he is consistently a joy to be around and he can be relied on to be around if needed.

And now, as an abrupt descent from all that exaltation, here I was on the road today with this same guy who's glowing over finding 22 cents in coins on the road yesterday and who's busily picking up coins today, trying to exceed yesterday's total loot. It's uncanny how the guy has radar for money on the road.

Dozens of times we've been on the road, side by side, and he's spotted coins unseen by me. From scholar to salvage, he does both with equal gusto.

Before starting today, I had resolved that along the way I would learn more about Paff's heart problem. I knew that in 1990 a cardiologist had diagnosed him with heart-muscle damage in three areas – a condition Paff called "silent ischemia."

I also knew the cardiologist had recommended a four-way bypass, but Paff balked at that saying he first wanted to try to correct the problem by modifying his lifestyle (diet, sleep, workload). And I knew for sure that subsequently Paff ran into a heap of troubles:

Along the way, he had to be "paddled" back to life three times, that he did have to submit to the operation and that he had complications from it.

To me – to any athlete – all this was damn serious stuff since this was a superb endurance athlete who had no previous signs of a heart condition. I wanted to know the whole sequence of events, the implications, the lessons, who's vulnerable (if he, why not me?) and anything else Paff thought appropriate to tell me.

All this in mind, I peppered him much of the day with questions to get this information. The story I learned read like this:

He said, "I went out for a casual walk in December 1993 – only one week after walking the Honolulu Marathon – and I suddenly and unexpectedly became light-headed. I sat down to rest and gather myself.

"I was sufficiently obtunded that I had no idea of what was happening. In fact, I was so confused that I wasn't able to think what could possibly be happening.

After 10 minutes or so I got up and started to make my way home, only two blocks away. Every 10 yards I had to rest.

"Arriving home, I took an aspirin and went to bed. I could not remember the 911 number.

"I did remember that Jo Ann would be home soon. She drove me to the hospital, where the process of getting my ventricular tachycardia back to a normal heartbeat started.

"Two hours later my heart beat was still 220 per minute. But a half-hour after that it was back to a normal 72.

"Some days later my regular cardiologist gave me an exercise-tolerance test, and I reached 13 on the Borg Scale. Then I stepped off the treadmill, took two steps and went into cardiac arrest. I had to be resuscitated.

"I revived, but shortly afterwards my heart stopped again. And again I was paddled back to life.

"The next move was to intensive care for four days and a workup for surgery. Thereafter, that didn't go too well. The complications after surgery were being back on a ventilator, convulsions, pulmonary emboli and bronchial pneumonia.

"All told I was in the hospital five weeks. After that my recovery was slow. It was six months before I was able to do daily walks of three miles."

As he talked, I kept thinking, How could this have happened to such a superb athlete?

Answering that, Paff said, "Well, I've already lived longer than any of the males in my mother's family. My presumption is that from her side of the family there is some genetic predisposition to a heart attack. But that's only speculation derived from ruling out the risk factors."

After the day's run Elaine was surprised not in the least when we asked her to stop at the ice cream shop and the bakery. "With you two it figures!" she said.

Good sport that she is, she even joined us for a double-decker cone as well as for an apple fritter. That's the top of the line in pit crewing!

DAY THREE. As we made the 48-mile drive from Kona to the start this morning, the same drive as yesterday afternoon after we'd finished, I was somewhat more knowledgeable of Route 19 than I had been three days prior. I had learned that 19 (which is the main drag from Hilo to Waimea and the west Kona coast of the island) goes by different names in different areas. It's the "Hawaii Belt Road" directly north of Hilo; it's the "Mamalahoa Highway" when it heads west from Honokaa for Waimea; it's "Kawaihae Road" when it goes from Waimea to Waiku (near Samuel M. Spencer Beach Park and junction of Highways 19/270); it's the Kawaiha Road" when it heads south from Waiku to Kailua-Kona. But not to worry; the road signs all along the way show it as Route 19.

When I imparted this information about the many faces of Route 19 to Elaine, she said, "You're always cramming your brain with needless information."

"Better that," I retorted, "than what Norman van Brocklin said about the brains of sports writers."

"Okay, I'm asking for it," she said. "But who was van Brocklin, and what did he say?"

"He was an NFL quarterback and he said something to the effect that if he ever had to have a brain transplant, he wanted one of a sports writer because it never would have been used."

We were about eight miles west of Waimea when we started, and we'd gone only a half-mile or so when we started downhill, which meant we were leaving the Waimea plateau.

For a few moments we were occupied with trying to analyze why

10 different homes all in a row, homes about a mile west that we saw yesterday and today, were for sale. The only tag we could put on it was their being on the wet side of the island.

I told Paff, "In the two years I lived on Oahu, I learned a little about buying real estate in Hawaii, but that's all fuzzy now. About all I can remember is that it is complicated with terms like 'fee simple' and 'leasehold.'

"Best as I can remember, 'fee simple' means you can pass the property to your heirs. 'Leasehold' means you own the property for the term of the lease, which can be as long as 99 years. I don't know about now, but back then, I'm talking 1963, it was hard to acquire 'fee simple' property."

"Considering the prices, it's hard to buy any desirable real estate in Hawaii," Paff noted.

Yesterday we'd seen a few horses and cows. Today they were more numerous. Lucky that this was a short day because Paff and I were getting weary from talking to so many of them.

The expression of the horses seemed to say, "Is that so?" Whereas those of the cows seemed to be, "Say what?"

As we edged into a setting of rolling hills and grass, and saw livestock scattered all about, I assumed all this was part of the Parker Ranch holding. Ye gods, with 225,000 acres, what wasn't?

A new critter came onto the scene today. Every so often as we'd see one dash across the highway, I was not sure whether we were looking at a mongoose or a weasel. I yelled, "Slow down so I can take a good look at you." They heeded me not at all.

One of the most impressionable sights of the day came around three miles when we saw two crosses roadside, one white and one blue. The white one was decorated with flowers and a string of beads, the blue one with a wreath and flowers.

On the fence behind the white one was a T-shirt with "Kokua" printed on it. Above "Kokua" were the words "Nation in distress" and below "Kokua" the words "Hawaiian nation." Evidently this was a cultural or political statement, one lost to me, I regretted.

On the fence behind the blue cross hung a T-shirt with a design showing a surfer. Nearby, leaning on the fence, was a tattered surf board.

So many crosses in so many states have I seen, and with each one arises the question: What caused this fatal accident? Though I've seen more than 100 highway crosses, that question has been answered only once – that being when I was told (in North Carolina, as I recall) that a 16-year old-girl driving on ice had rolled her car.

One pleasant aspect of the day was having the warm sun radiating to my ancient bones and renewing their energy, or so it felt to me. Contrarily Elaine was bemoaning the hot weather. As for Paff, heat or cold, little matter – he was a man on a mission and success, not weather, was material.

Actually success was easy to come by today, this being only a 6.5-mile day. Around 5.6 miles we left Route 19, turned east and headed down Paakalau Street toward downtown Honokaa.

Once we hit the main street of this town of 2000 souls, two words came immediately to mind, "quaint" and "sleepy" – even though this is the biggest town on the Hamakua coast. Most of the shops seemed to specialize in Hawaiian products and crafts.

We had not wandered in Honokaa very long before I realized I'd not done my homework very well. I had expected that from town it would be a simple stroll to the ocean, slightly east. But as we made several forays trying to get to the ocean, we kept encountering fences and "No Trespassing" signs.

In today's world, realizing that we could be invading a marijuana field – fields often protected by aggressive owners with guns – Paff and I entertained no notions of heading through private property to get to the ocean. Yet the ocean was where I wanted to finish. As John Masefield said in his poem "Sea Fever":

> *I must go down to the seas again*
> *for the call of the running tide*
> *Is a wild call and a clear call*
> *that may not be denied.*

Groping for a way to get to the ocean, we made inquiries of five people but answers from only three – two natives and a storekeeper. The question we asked was, "What is the shortest way to get to the ocean from town?" We got three different answers.

One native simply said there was no place around Honokaa where we could get to the ocean, and the other native said that maybe the closest place was Samuel Spencer Beach, where we had started our venture two days before. The storekeeper said the closest spot was Keokea Beach Park.

My reaction was to look at a map to locate Keokea Beach. It turned out to be on the northern end of the island, about 40 miles away.

The situation was serious. We decided that the only strategy was to discuss it over lunch.

That in mind we descended on Jolene's Kau Kau Club (yes, I did a double-take with "kau kau" and felt better when I learned it's Hawaiian slang for food).

Two good things came out of Jolene's: First, the saimin was delicious. But better yet the young waitress was able to answer our question about ocean access. The only downside to this was we felt we had to double her tip

"The closest place to get to the ocean," she told us, "is Waipio State Beach. It's straight north up Route 240. I'd guess it's about nine miles to the beach."

Nine miles! Tilt!

That was my first thought. We were scheduled to depart Hawaii tomorrow, and no way would Elaine and I allow Paff another nine miles today despite his probably being willing to try it.

I mulled the problem momentarily. And as I did, two thoughts unfolded:

1. If I wanted to get to the ocean, I had only one alternative – return to Hawaii later and finish those nine miles.
2. If I could save those nine miles until after I'd completed the other 49 states, I could finish Hawaii as the 50th state. Thus was born the idea of making Hawaii our 50th state to finish.

Turning to Elaine and Paff, I said, "Since we're leaving tomorrow, I don't see any way out of this except to return here later and do the nine miles to the ocean. I kind of like the idea of returning here and finishing Hawaii as the 50th state. Some dramatic value there."

"Good idea," Paff said. "I second it. Count me in."

But not Elaine. "Well," she replied, "think of it as a drama without me. You've already crossed Hawaii, and I'm not coming again. Besides, I don't get along with this Hawaii heat."

I felt that Elaine would change her mind. I also felt negligent in not doing my homework and learning that Waipio State Beach Park was the closest ocean access.

On the other hand I very much liked the idea of finishing Hawaii as the 50th state. I figured we'd most likely do that in December since Paff habitually comes to Oahu during the Honolulu Marathon week in December, when he talks at the American Medical Athletic Association annual conference.

Hearing Elaine led me to change the subject abruptly – or maybe astutely since I decided Elaine did not appreciate the decision of Hawaii as the 50th state. I said to Paff, "Well, how does it feel to have lunch with the riffraff?"

He looked at me quizzically, and before he could answer I went on, "I mean that at the International Olympic Committee awards luncheon you sat besides Princess Anne of Great Britain, and a couple of months ago you had lunch with Prince Albert of Monaco, Prince Alexandre de Merode of Belgium and President Juan Antonio Samaranch of the IOC. Now you're having lunch with us peasants."

"True," Paff said, "but just think what the princess and princes are missing by not enjoying this saimin. Royalty has its price."

Reviewing Hawaii, the best as I could calculate we'd logged between 25.8 and 26.0 miles in our three-day stroll across the island. I almost felt abnormal in being able to derive so much pleasure out of this simple outing.

I also felt good to see Paff enjoying himself. With his schedule the guy deserves all the R&R he can squeeze in.

Paff and I were already looking forward to the last nine miles in December. Not so Elaine.

"I've heard you quote Samuel Goldwyn several times before," she said. "You know, his 'Include me out' words.

"That's me on this nine-mile thing. It's dumb. You have already crossed Hawaii!"

John Masefield, what do you say to that?

DAY FOUR. Jumping ahead to December 11th, the logistics of getting to the start of our long-delayed fourth and final day in Hawaii were cluttered – consisting of the drive from our Oahu hotel to the airport, the 6:30 A.M. flight from Honolulu to Kona, then the drive from Kona to the hamlet of Honokaa', the starting point.

Actually Paff and I had the luxury of being passengers all the way because his wife, Jo Ann, made all the arrangements and did all the driving. Jo Ann, a nurse practitioner, even volunteered to pit crew for us and had rented a Buick Skylark for the occasion.

Accompanied by an MD and a nurse practitioner, I was in good hands. If ever I were to get ill or injured on the road, the time should be now, with immediate medical aid at hand.

Paff and I were eager to get the show on the road as we debarked in Honokaa – a sleepy hamlet of 2000 souls, quaint old buildings and stores featuring mainly native products. The day was cool by Hawaii standards – low 70s, a bit windy, cloudy, considerably kinder to walking/running than our three previous days on the island had been.

"I guarantee it won't rain," Jo Ann told us as we started. She based her forecast on having lived in the islands for 27 years, 1961 to 1988.

Our route was northward along Highway 240, a two-lane road with a bike lane on both sides. Lightly traveled and quite comfortable.

A short distance out of town we came across a cemetery on the west side of the road with two unusual aspects: All the inscriptions were in Japanese, and it was located on a steep terraced hill.

The next attraction, this about a half-mile into our day, was the Mauna Kea Physical Therapy building. We logged that for future use in case the going got rough.

A short way up the road we saw Jo Ann standing roadside with camera in hand. "I want to take your picture in front of that lava tube," she told us. The huge cave, on the west side of the road, was located adjacent to the highway.

Well, here we go again, I thought. Another one of dozens of pictures with this Paffenbarger guy, who always looks so much more dynamic than I in photos.

By now both Paff and I were noticing that the vegetation and foliage were considerably greener than when we'd been here in February. So far, all along the route a steep hill was to our left, the west, and on our right, the east, was a descent to the ocean a mile or so away. Grass and coniferous trees covered the descent side, and sugar cane was common on the ascent side.

The modest homes scattered along the route were all fugitives from any painting. Almost all of them had corrugated tin roofs.

All along the way we were seeing typical Hawaiian flora – hibiscus, poinsettias, bougainvillea. Most of the time we had a sweeping view of the ocean.

"You guys are sure doing a lot of chatting," we heard Jo Ann say at one of the early pit stops. True.

One new wrinkle in our conversation was Paff talked about the dog he and Jo Ann had recently acquired. For years Jo Ann had been lobbying for a dog, and Paff had stalled by saying, "Maybe tomorrow."

When he surrendered a couple months ago and they acquired a Boston terrier, they named him "Morgen" – which, so I learned, is German for tomorrow.

Several times as we went down the road today Paff gave me reports on Morgen. He stopped just short of waving a portfolio of pictures of Morgen. He might have balked at getting a dog, but now he is 100-percent smitten.

Around 2.5 miles I stopped to take a picture of Waipio B&B Inn. Doing so, I thought this was a foolish maneuver since I had no use whatsoever for the photo.

When we passed the road leading to Kapulena Orchards around four miles, I had to restrain Paff from making a reconnaissance to check on the products. Could be there were no products since the place posted a Pacific Realty for-sale sign.

A good feeling it was to see Paff so perked up. Ye gods, only four days earlier the guy had returned home after a 23-hour flight from South Africa.

Jo Ann shared my observation of Paff because at the five-mile pit stop she commented, "I'm glad to see you looking so frisky today."

She was pampering us by stopping every mile where we'd have a short visit and something to eat and drink. Nutritionist Covert Bailey would endorse the purism of our sticking with water, but he would frown at the cookies and candies.

As we went along, I was basking in the luxury of the easy pace, a brisk walk and the pleasure of good company. But I did miss sharing with Elaine who had been with me for 557 other days on the road.

Crossing two bridges (built in 1963 and 1972, juveniles compared to Paff and me), we took time out to observe the water cascading over the huge rocks in the streams below. The Waipuaho Stream bordered on being a waterfall.

At one point along the way Paff jumped with jubilation when he found a penny, thus keeping intact his record of finding money each of our four days across Hawaii.

A little past four miles when we came to a split in the road – the left sign reading Waipio, the right Kukuihaele – I was uncertain which road to follow. Dr. "Livingstone" Paffenbarger proclaimed that we should go right.

Doing so, we soon came to the Last Chance Store that sells groceries, gas and sundries. So well stocked from one-mile pit stops were we that we were not tempted to buy any goodies.

From the quick glance I had I deduced that the adjacent Waipio Valley Art Works dealt only in quality products. I also deduced that we were in the Kukuihaele area though there were no signs to that effect.

At times, as Paff moved along at a brisk walk, I found myself having to jog to keep up with him – quite understandable since my walking pace sometimes seems to be one step short of rigor mortis.

All along the way Paff and I kept up a constant conversation. I was anxious to hear about the four trips he had made in the past two months while talking in Japan, Monaco, South Africa and Orlando. I was envious of his Japan trip because he got to visit Kyoto, something I was not able to do during the 14 months I lived in the country and was occupied with Marine Corps duties not permitting the travel time.

I asked if he had run on the prince's private all-weather track in Monaco, and he replied, "I didn't even get to see it."

We talked about our mutual friend in South Africa, Tim Noakes – an MD who is world famous in sports medicine. His book *The Lore of Running* could well be the best book ever written about distance running.

We talked about the recent, unexpected death of one of his colleagues, Bob Hyde of Alcoa, Tennessee. A death that like those of other close friends made both of us feel, without ever saying it, that we were one step closer to our graves, that great divide.

Talking, observing the scenery, we found ourselves sooner than expected at the next landmark, the Waipio Valley overlook. This is the takeoff point for the steep descent – 1000 feet in one mile – to the floor of the Waipio Valley. Only four-wheeled vehicles are allowed on the one-mile paved road.

Jo Ann had parked the car and was ready to make the descent into the valley with us. This would be a leisurely stroll for her, an athlete who had won the women's division of the first 100-kilometer race in

Honolulu and who finished the 36-mile Run to the Sun race (which goes from sea level to the peak of Haleokala at 10,000 feet) on Maui the same year I ran it. On this jaunt I considered her a walking paramedic!

We paused at the overlook to stare at the valley, verdant green and about one mile across. We stood atop the south ridge.

The north ridge was an even steeper pali. We could see the entire one-mile length of the ocean beach, the longest in Hawaii, as it pounded onto the black sand extending between the two ridges.

The river, the Waipio, flowing through the valley and into the ocean, was clearly visible. Not visible was Waipio Waterfalls, located at the head of the valley and masked by the ridge on which we stood.

Bong! was our first reaction as we started down the paved road into the valley. Damn thing seemed straight down, certainly the steepest paved road I've ever been on.

Judging from the eight-percent gradient I often drive near my home, I judged this gradient to be 25 to 30 percent. Gotta write to the Hawaiian Highway Department and find out, I told myself.

We had to brace ourselves as we went down. Running here would be to invite disaster.

Several times – well, eight to be exact, – we had to step aside for vehicles. We either hugged the guard rail or the cliff.

Well aware that there have been 20 fatalities on this one-mile stretch, we were extremely cautious. Which was somewhat understandable in that none of us wanted to become number 21.

After a mile down the steep, paved road we came to a dirt road going straight ahead and a muddy road to the right, a 180 degrees from our down direction. Seeing no signs, and confused about the shortest distance to the beach, we elected to go straight. In a half-mile or so we got a good view of Waipio Waterfalls at the head of the valley.

As we were studying the falls, a native in a pickup came by. From him we learned that to get to the ocean we should have taken the muddy road near the end of the paved downhill.

We retreated and made our way to the ocean, The muddy road, with trees and foliage to its very edges, hugged the bottom of the valley's south pali.

The distance from the end of the paved road to the ocean was only a half-mile or so. By the time we reached the ocean, we had covered 10 miles for the day, and we still had 1.5 miles to do to get back to the car – mileage not counted as part of my state crossings.

Arriving at the ocean, the first thing I noticed was that the entire beach was lined with rocks – most of them football or basketball size, and extending from the ocean about 10 feet or more onto the beach. Next I took note of the size and natural raw beauty of the sandy beach that extended inland a hundred or more yards. A few camping signs, widely separated, were posted on trees, and they represented the only home improvements in the entire area.

I found myself regretting that we did not have time to explore the entire valley, to get to the base of the falls, to walk across the valley floor. Here, not Waikiki, was the true Hawaii.

I knew little about the valley, never having been here before. I had read that it was capable of producing enough foodstuffs to feed the entire populace of the island. I had read about a bare-basics hotel operating in the valley and that these days only about 50 people lived in the valley.

The next move was a photo session. In one shot I was heading into the ocean, soaking and abusing my shoes that had served me so faithfully.

As I stood in the water, my thoughts went back to dipping my toes in the Atlantic at Hilton Head Island, South Carolina, upon finishing the USA run. Never did I realize then, after crossing 12 states, that I'd subsequently go on to run across the other 38.

On finishing the USA run, I was bubbly with excitement – high because of the achievement. A feeling shared by Elaine.

Today, by contrast, was low-keyed as I stood in awe of the scenery and setting while being quietly overwhelmed with the realization that after 7646.5 miles of foot travel, 558 days on the road (353 of them spent running), 60,000 miles of motorhome driving by Elaine, air trips to Florida, Alaska and Hawaii, and 500 miles of rented cars, the final chapter was now written in our odyssey of 50 states.

Elaine had been with me – hell, had ministered unto me – all but the last 10 of those miles. I sorely missed sharing with her today. I much wanted to stand at the water's edge with her, arms around each other – just as we had done at Hilton Head – and share the moment with her.

I was glad that Paff and Jo Ann were about. By myself it would have been a very lonely moment.

I guess I must be what teenagers these days call "a square," for here I was having a ball by simply walking, talking and enjoying beautiful scenery with a couple of close friends. Waipio Valley, for me, would be an experience remembered unto death.

Leaving the beach, I stopped momentarily to talk with Tom Harrington, a San Francisco resident who said he owns some property in the valley area. "What you must do someday," he said, "is walk across the valley. You'll have to ford a few small streams on the way, but it's worth it when you get to the other side and experience the beauty of walking on a path of flowers and hachens under an umbrella of banyan trees."

When I told him we would have liked to get closer to the falls, he replied, "Well, at one time this was a twin waterfall. But either the Parker Ranch or the sugar-cane people, I don't know which, covered one of the canals feeding the falls and this resulted in having only one waterfall. The canal was supposed to be restored, but that never has happened."

At one point during the arduous ascent up the steep paved road I asked Paff, "Is this how it felt when you ran into trouble on that walk in 1993?"

"Not even close," Paff replied. "By comparison, this is all downhill."

To celebrate the occasion, Paff and I decided we would return to Jolene's Cafe in Honokaa and have saimin for lunch – just as we had done after finishing our first three days in Hawaii. But on this score we met defeat, as contrasted with our victorious day, because Jolene's was closed. As any coach will tell you, "Can't win em all."

Oh Lord, how the human mind works. As we were driving back to the Kona airport, I found myself thinking, Now that I've done all 50 states, what's next? Like the man said, always have an agenda if you want to stay young at heart.

Flying from Kona to Honolulu and seated apart form Paff and Jo Ann, I reviewed the entire business of running across all 50 states from those first steps out of the Pacific Ocean, at Jenner, California, on April 20th, 1990, to the final steps today at Waipio Valley, Hawaii, on December 11th, 1997.

The time lapse was 2780 days, 353 of which I had been on the road. Almost an entire year of my life being a roads scholar. Ditto for Elaine – her being cook, chauffeur, nurse, chaplain, companion, confidante, pit crew and rooting section.

Together we had lived a dream, and our odyssey had enriched our lives. The sharing had bonded us closer together.

We had built a reservoir of memories, a portfolio of lessons learned. Working together, we had met the challenge; we succeeded in doing what no one else has ever done.

Along the way we came to appreciate and understand more of this vast and great country of ours. It had been a great ride, a joyful journey, one made, by the grace of God, without injury or illness to either of us.

And now, as the plane was about to land in Honolulu airport, I started to think, Well, it's over. But as I did so, my mind flashed back to the day we finished our USA run and we were standing at the ocean's edge at Hilton Head Island, South Carolina.

I asked Elaine, "What are you thinking?"

She replied, "That it's over – and yet it will never really be over. It's something that will always be with us, a part of us – just yours and mine."

I found myself chuckling when, out of the blue and in answer to her, a phrase popular during my Marine Corps tour of duty in Japan came to mind: "You better Hong Kong well believe!"

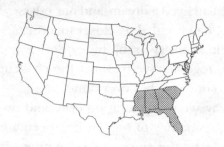

Mississippi, Alabama, Georgia, South Carolina and Florida

The Rest of the Story

Mississippi, Alabama, Georgia and South Carolina were four of the 12 states crossed during our USA run in 1990. Our adventures across each of these states are described in four full chapters, one per state, in the book *Ten Million Steps*. The runs across each of these states are summarized below. I also report on a separate 1996 run across Florida so that this book will include a complete accounting of all the 26 states east of the Mississippi River: the 21 run in 1997, the four run in 1990 and the one run in 1996.

Mississippi

Dates: *July 23rd to 30th, 1990*

Miles: *178.3*

Route: *Start in Helena, Arkansas, on Highway 49. Follow 49 east to Highway 61, cross 61 and take Highway 315 east to I-55. Cross I-55 and follow 310 east to 340, then continue to 340 south to Highway 78/30. Take 30 to its junction with Highway 9 to where it joins Highway 4, continue on 4 to Highway 25, which goes south to Alabama border.*

Mississippi began on a lively note when I was told that the Helena police were tied up in court and unable to provide an escort for me across the bridge over the Mississippi River. "You'll have to negotiate it by yourself," they said.

Arriving at the bridge and seeing no cars approaching from the left lane, I busted my butt running the bridge hill and got two-thirds of the way before the first cars appeared.

I stopped, hugged the bridge rail and waited until they passed, ran again until reaching a 12-inch ledge – almost a sidewalk – that ran the length of the center span. Then I ran on the road whenever possible and jumped to the ledge as cars drew close.

After the last car went through the stoplight at the end of the bridge, I took off as fast as I could before the light turned loose another flock of cars. I knew damn well that this all-out effort would cost me dearly as the miles mounted later in the day.

But I was triumphant, reaching the highway just as the first car started up the bridge. Elaine's crossing was nerve-wracking, too, because the one lane on the bridge was barely wide enough to accommodate the motorhome.

After a short while in the state I made a couple of sociological notes. All through Kansas, Missouri, Oklahoma, Arkansas and now Mississippi, I've seen laundry on clotheslines. That is rarely seen these days in California.

At an early pit stop Elaine noted the negative way that folks here ask questions. She'd had two offers of help when parked here. The exact words were, "Y'all aren't broken down, are you?" and "Y'all don't need any help, do you?"

I got a sample when a fellow asked, "You ain't in trouble, are you?"

By now, beginning our 94th day on the road when entering Mississippi, Elaine, alone in the motorhome when I was on the road, was getting lonesome – to the point where she asked me to find a turtle as company for her. So I went on turtle patrol and, having scouted 30 or more ponds and creeks, have not yet found a single turtle. (I'm inclined to add, probably from being on the road too long, and that I haven't spotted a a married one either.)

At one pit stop I teased Elaine by saying, "I saw this small turtle, and I asked him, 'Do you want to go to South Carolina?' He said, 'Git away from me, skinny ol' white man!' "

As I moved through Mississippi, several unanswered questions came up:

1. I went past church after church, most of them nice brick buildings. How can such a sparse population with no apparent signs of wealth support so many churches?

2. In an area with so few people, I passed by a place with six large moving vans parked out front. Who (okay, WHOM) do they move?

3. Amid generally low-quality, low-cost housing I occasionally saw what could only be described as a mansion. Why would someone who could afford to build such a home choose to put it here?

4. Throughout Mississippi, as in some other southern states, I've noticed that dumpsters are placed at various road junctions for deposit of garbage. Why then are Mississippi roads strewn with more litter than any state I've seen?

Two major nuisances in Mississippi have been flies and mosquitoes. Big horse flies, and when I say "big," I mean about the size of a grasshopper.

I've battled mosquitoes in Alaska, the Solomon Islands and North Carolina, but never so many as have hit us some mornings here. First question on my mind as I hit the road most mornings was, "How hungry are the mosquitoes today?"

Speaking of insects, at one pit stop Elaine showed me a one-inch by two-inch hole in the fiberglass screen on our motorhome window. She explained, "I was sitting in the dining area, heard this noise by the screen, and looked up to see some huge insect devouring the fiberglass."

She doused him with Raid and patched the screen with duct tape. That was her excitement for the day.

There were several amusing experiences in Mississippi. One happened when I stopped in Sardis for a haircut. Doing so in this small town reminded me of a scene in the movie "Treasure of the Sierra Madre" in which Humphrey Bogart goes into a barber shop in a small Mexican town and comes out with a weird bowl haircut.

I wondered, Will I meet the same fate in Sardis?. First surprise, the barber was a woman. Second surprise, outstanding haircut – a barber in the Biltmore Hotel could not have done better. Some days you just live right!

Then there was the day when I attracted almost as many curiosity-seekers as mosquitoes. It started when Elaine, parked at a pit stop, told some people there about our run.

When I came along, they were all standing there to see the 73-year-old man who runs. So it has come to this?

And it didn't end there, because two encores followed. Three miles later another half-dozen folks had gathered, yes, to see this 73-year-old weirdo who runs.

The second encore came about when three guys wanted, in their words, "to see what the 73-year-old wonder boy looks like." I was beginning to feel like an oddity.

The climax to all this came when Elaine and I were enjoying a snack in the motorhome and the three guys returned with a friend. He opened the screen door, stuck his head in and said, "I just got to see what you look like!"

As I had the habit of doing throughout the USA run, I made several assessments of aches and pains. I philosophized that if I ran into trouble, it would first be joints, second because of bones, third because of tendons and fourth because of muscles.

The farther I get into this USA run (days 94 through 100 were in Mississippi), the more tired became muscles, tendons and bones, and the more apprehensive I became when a problem appeared. I was afraid it could develop into the collapse of a working body component, and then I'd be in big trouble.

A thought kept crossing my mind, one I can't express too often or too emphatically: On a trek like this the runner's got to believe–believe he can keep going, believe he'll make it to the end, believe that doing it serves a worthwhile purpose.

We weakened one night in Mississippi and stayed in a motel, the Hallmark Inn in Albany, for the kind price of $29.95. More attractive than the price in the unbearably hot weather was the air conditioning, not available in the motorhome because there were no RV parks in the vicinity with electrical hookups.

Generally speaking, though, Mississippi's state parks were available and usually had RV hookups. The only state park where we had trouble was the Elvis Presley State Park.

Trouble on two counts: First, our start was delayed 45 minutes when we had to wait for a ranger to show up and unlock the gate.

(Interesting attire when he did show: shoeless, ball cap, swimming trunks.) Second count, Elvis, who's appeared to so many people, failed to make the scene.

Traveling on unmarked back roads, we got lost a couple of times in Mississippi, but someone was always around to point us in the right direction. I particularly remembered one high school kid, out skateboarding at daybreak, who gave us excellent directions.

While we had no major problems, we did have a few unpleasant incidents. Typical was the one near our finish when four teenagers in the back of a pickup threw some firecrackers at me and enjoyed seeing me jump.

Demonstrating superb restraint, I did not salute them with an obscene gesture. Come to think of it, maybe it wasn't restraint, maybe I was just too tired.

On the plus side of the ledger, most of the drivers were courteous and considerate. All the people Elaine and I talked with were upbeat and we shared a number of laughs.

All told, Mississippi was a pleasant experience.

Alabama

Dates: *July 30th to August 6th, 1990*
Miles: *181.7*
Route: *Start at Mississippi/Alabama border on Highway 24 at Red Bay and follow 24 to its junction with Highway 36. East on 36 to junction with 231. At 231 take Highway 66 east to 431. At 431 follow Highway 75 to its junction with Highway 35 and continue on 35 east to Georgia border.*

Our approach to most of the small towns seen coming across the USA has been through a corridor of residences. Not so with Alabama and the city of Red Bay. We were into heavy business development immediately.

From all the action, including an Allegro motorhome plant, I surmised that the local economy is good. As for Red Bay it was so-named, I assumed, because the soil in this area is the same type of red clay that I've seen in places as diverse as Georgia, Guam and Placerville, California.

Our entry into Alabama was not too encouraging in that the only day of bad weather we experienced during seven days in the state happened out first day when we were in a thunderstorm and heavy rain for six miles. Actually, though, being wet is not as uncomfortable as being hot – especially with the humidity. The major problem with rain is the damage it does to shoes.

One of the scariest mornings we had on the USA crossing happened when we were at Bear Creek Reservoir Campground. We were up shortly after four A.M. and at 4:20 heard a knock on the motorhome door.

"Yes," I called. Two more knocks in the predawn darkness.

"What do you want?" I shouted. Hesitation, then, "I have a memorandum for you from the camp commander."

This sounded phony. First, the camp commander had told us all we needed to know.

Second, what reasonable person would be sending a memo at four in the morning? I didn't like this, especially since we were isolated from other campers.

I replied, "We don't need it," and waited for the knocker's next move.

"Okay," he said, then walked to his car and drove off. By my reckoning what he really wanted us to do was to open the door to the motorhome.

After a short while in Alabama, I noticed that most of the men drivers waved when they spotted me. The women didn't. They're paralyzed with the thought, "What's this old coot doing out here in his BVD's?"

The first person I talked with in Alabama was a state trooper, a black officer. He asked, "Are you just out for exercise?"

I explained the task at hand and what our M.O is. The trooper was a bright young man with a degree in business administration.

"Before joining the Highway Patrol," he said, "I worked in an office but didn't like the confinement. I like the work I'm doing now because it gets me out and lets me meet people."

I asked him a number of questions, and I didn't like one answer he gave when I asked about snakes. "There are rattlers, copperheads, and water moccasins about," he said. Just the kind of news I needed.

One of the main dangers on the road, especially around Red Bay, was that many 14-foot-wide mobile homes were being towed. I measured the road and found it to be not quite 11 feet from the white fog line to the center of the road. Most of the truck drivers seeing one of these mobile homes approaching moved to the outside of the road – something I had in common with these drivers except that I fled to the hinterlands.

As was her habit on the USA run, Elaine would park some mornings then jog back to run a mile or so with me. One morning we got a scare when a hare-brained woman in a Cadillac, passing a truck and seeing us only as she was upon us, came within six inches of hitting us. A goose-pimple experience.

We ran into a logistical problem in Alabama some nights when there was not an RV park with hookups within 25 or more miles of where we finished. On one such night we decided to drive into Russellville and tap our motel budget to the tune of $31.50 at the Village Inn.

In a spending mood we dined – maybe not elegantly but at least enjoyably – at the Pizza Hut. Hey, that Veggie Lover's pan pizza was ammunition for the next day's run.

Another night we drove into Hartselle to scout for an RV hookup, found none and decided to live dangerously – and economically. We parked for the night in a shopping center lot.

Hartselle won our award for the outstanding town on our route. It definitely had personality.

Its four-block business section had a metal awning covering all the store fronts, making this sort of an outdoor mall. The wrought iron decorating the awning reflected history.

By contrast Danville did not appear to be the finest of communities.

Going through the state, I could not help but notice some of the unusual names of different Baptist churches" Burn Out Baptist Church, Highway 36 Baptist Church, Ironman Baptist Church, just to name a few.

At times I was entertained by watching a farm operation, like the farmer with a tractor pulling a cutter/thresher. The machine cut a row of corn stalks, picked them up and deposited them in a mulcher, which then dumped them in a truck for use as cattle feed.

One of the most memorable strips of roadway was the causeway leading into Guntersville. I came upon a crane standing on a rock beside the lake, and it took off as I came near, skimming over the water. Never before have I been able to look down on a flying crane like this, and it had a beautiful flight pattern.

Thirty ducks nearby swam farther out into the lake. In the distant east I saw heavily forested mountains.

At the east edge of the causeway I saw that the city has an attractive recreational complex, bordered by a lake and forest. Viewing this new scenery, instead of farm after farm, added an air of adventure and excitement.

Highway 35 from Rainsville to Fort Payne was bumper-to-bumper housing. Some homes were residential, and some sat on farms so small they could be called "backyard" farms.

Nearing Fort Payne, I went down a long, steep hill on a road so narrow there was no shoulder, just a drop down a ledge. From the top of the hill I saw nothing but mountains. Fort Payne lay in a narrow valley, so there was no way out except by crossing those mountains.

Fort Payne has a long history. The fort was built by order of General Winfield Scott and named after a Captain John Payne, who was stationed here. It dates from 1848.

Some of the present town reflects this history. The town also lays claim to Sequoyah, an Indian genius who conceived and perfected (over a 12-year period) an alphabet of 84 letters.

Because of this alphabet, most of the Cherokee nation could read and write. The giant Sequoia trees and Sequoia National Park were named in his honor, though not staying true to the spelling of the chief's name.

Fort Payne was our closest brush with history in Alabama.

Georgia

Dates: *August 6th to 18th, 1990*
Miles: *321.2*
Route: *Start at Alabama/Georgia border on Highway 48, follow 48 east to Highway 27. South to Highway 140, then 140 east to Highways 19/120, and 120 east to Highways 311/20, then 20 southeast to Highways 78/83. Follow 83 south to 129/278, and 278 east to I-80/80. Take 80 east to 121/24, and 24 south to Highway 23, Follow 23 southeast to Highway 301 and take 301 across Savannah River into South Carolina.*

Near the Alabama/Georgia border as we saw the first signs advertising boiled peanuts, I concluded we must be in Jimmy Carter territory. At the next pit stop beside a general store, guess who was sitting in the motorhome munching boiled peanuts when I arrived. Elaine reported, "They taste somewhat like beans."

One of the first sights to catch my eye in Georgia was a cemetery with a large monument reading "Reese." A little spooky to see my name on a tombstone, especially as tired as I was.

Our first night in Georgia, finishing near Summerville, we gained respect for the Georgia state park system when we stayed at James H. Floyd State Park. It had excellent facilities and was spotlessly clean.

Looking back over 100 days, Elaine and I agreed that about the biggest disappointment of the trip has been the little recreational time we get after the running is done. By the time we locate an RV place, have our showers, have dinner, I do my writing and Elaine does her chores, and then check the routing and camping possibilities for the next day, it's bedtime.

Sometimes while trying to hold myself together, I felt like a pilot going over a checklist: (1) Is the sacroiliac belt fastened tightly? (2) Need any Aspercreme? (3) How about suntan lotion? (4) Blistex – got some on? (5) Water bottle filled? (6) Injury assessment? (7) Carrying repellent for mosquitoes and chiggers?

One of the most distressing sights on the road has been the hundreds of animals killed on the highways. What bothers me most here is that most of these deaths are more the fault of drivers than of the animals.

I discovered that poultry farming is big in this area. I saw several farms with hundreds of chickens, all huddled together.

Some of the poultry sheds are close to the road. Believe me, they're odoriferous.

These sheds are 100 or more yards long with tin roofs, doors at each end and screened sides. Each shed has a couple of grain bins that pump feed to the birds inside.

A farmer told me, "One shed can house as many as 17,000 chickens."

In Waleska I went past Rinehard College, which was founded in 1883. I got the impression that it stresses academics and doubt if it even has a football team; I know that it's not on Notre Dame's schedule. About the only distraction in this hamlet for students is a convenience store.

My friend Frank Bacon, a retired Marine Corps colonel, had forewarned us, "If you get anywhere near Atlanta, the traffic will snow you under."

We did, and it did. The drivers displayed the discourteous big-city mentality.

The commute traffic was heavily sprinkled with BMWs and Mercedes. Seeing them, I thought, "If I'm going to get hit, let it be by one of these rich dudes or dames."

The suburban area of Atlanta, particularly Alpharette, reeked of affluence. What I did not understand was why – with all the affluence in the area – were the roads so dangerously narrow?

An incident in Georgia was as close as I came to a confrontation during the entire USA run. It began when three guys in a pickup, trying to scare me, veered off the road and into the weeds, heading straight toward me.

To escape I ran farther into the weeds, and as they went past, one of them banged the metal door of the pickup. This caused me to jump, arousing my Marine Corps fighting blood, and I gave them the European obscene gesture.

That, I thought, was the end of it. But about three minutes later they returned, and one of the guys got out of the pickup and yelled, "You gave me the finger!"

Trying to placate him, I shouted back, "Sorry about the gesture, but you scared the hell out of me." Then I realized the guy bordered on being drunk.

He surprised me by saying, "If I had seen how old you are, I wouldn't have done that."

We talked a bit, and finally he said, "Okay, let's shake hands and be friends."

After we shook hands, he insisted on hugging me and again told he how sorry he was. I now realized this guy was blotto. He wanted to hug me a couple more times, and I worried he might want to kiss.

Finally I yelled to the other two guys in the truck, "You'd better get him out of here, or people will be talking about us."

After he left, I smiled over this experience. After all, he could have come back with a shotgun or a .38. Visions of "Easy Rider" passed through my mind.

A meeting with three ladies in a Cadillac was more on the amusing side. They said they wanted to do a newspaper interview, so I answered a few questions and then told them they could get more details from Elaine who was parked a couple of miles down the road.

With southern elegance, one of them said, "We're honored to have you run through out town." A second added, not too diplomatically, "Especially at your age!"

When I caught up with Elaine, she reported that the women had a bet among them about my age. One of them had said, "He'll never see 70 again." That didn't help my self-image.

In Georgia as in other states I tried to get my mind off running by disassociating, dwelling on things other than the act of running. A good example of disassociating was reviewing my overriding impressions of the 11 states we'd passed through to this point.

California: the excitement of starting at Jenner, the sendoff by friends who ran the Slice 100 Km race with us, the snow at Carson Pass.

Nevada: the beautiful sunrises and sunsets of the desert, the surprise of so many mountains over 6000 feet elevation.

Utah: the caring people, the spectacular colors in the mountains.

Colorado: the majestic peaks, the many clear streams, the white water of the Arkansas River.

Kansas: the wheat fields and harvesting, the friendly people.

Oklahoma: the need for improvement on many counts.

Missouri: the surprising beauty of the Ozarks, more friendly people.

Arkansas: more of the Ozark Mountains and their enchantment.

Mississippi: the poverty of some of its people, the elation of running over the Mississippi River.

Alabama: the cotton and soybean fields.

Georgia: the miserable road and traffic conditions near Atlanta, the thick forestation.

On our ninth day in Georgia, Elaine and I were enjoying a snack at a pit stop when a car pulled up nearby. We saw two men walking toward us.

It took me a moment to see they weren't strangers. One was Frank Bacon who lives nearby in Milledgeville. He and his brother Paul had come out to welcome us to their state.

Frank and I were in the same Marine Corps officers' class, and we were both commissioned second lieutenants in January 1942. Frank's whole purpose in driving out here was to visit with us and to invite us to meet him and his wife, Margie, for dinner in Thompson the following evening.

As Frank drove off, Elaine and I felt our spirits elevated by his visit. That's a customary role for Frank, bringing joy to people.

He's president of our 7th ROC association, and as a result of his efforts a group of surviving classmates get together every year for a reunion. It's quite emotional to visit classmates you've known since 1942 – men who, like you, speak the language of World War II, the Marine Corps dialect.

As the days wind down, I reflect more and more on the countless things Elaine has done to ease the run for me. Never before has anyone been beside me over so long a period of time with us both zeroed in on accomplishing the same goal. Our togetherness and harmony brings me more pleasure than anything on this trip.

Several people have asked me, "How are you able to do 26 miles day after day?" I'm not sure whether they're thinking about the distance or my age, but I've yet to give a serious answer to that question. I usually dismiss it with a joking remark like, "One step at a time."

The serious answer, I guess, has something to do with mindset – the desire, dedication, determination to just do it, believing I can, hanging in there each day, giving no thought to quitting.

Near the end of our Georgia crossing and in the course of a pit-stop conversation, I asked Elaine, "What has been the toughest thing on the whole trip for you? You know what mine was, finding running space on the road."

Without hesitation, she replied, "The heat." That surprised me. I had expected her to say, "Finding a place to park the motorhome for pit stops."

As for heat, no doubt we made a major mistake in not getting a motorhome with a generator to keep it cool while Elaine was parked and waiting.

On our next to last day both Elaine and I got a laugh out of a conversation with a boy named Nicky. We had seen a crop we could not identify, and when we came upon 12-year-old Nicky we asked him about the crop – which he identified as peas.

In the course of the conversation we learned that the zenith of his life is visiting the Dairy Queen in Waynesboro. He also told us about a "great place" in Girard to get a Coke. Nicky's rotund shape testified that he was a frequent visitor to both places.

By the time we were edging out of Georgia and completing more than 3100 miles, I felt as if I could almost smell the Atlantic, our finish, about 90 miles away. Elaine and I were eager to invade South Carolina, and head for Hilton Head Island and the Atlantic.

South Carolina

Dates: *August 18th to 22nd, 1990*
Miles: *87.5*
Route: *Start at Georgia/South Carolina border on bridge over Savannah River on Highway 301, go east to Highway 601, then south on 601 to its junction with Highway 652. Follow 652 southeast to I-95 and Highway 278. Take 278 southeast to Hilton Head Island and, arriving there, follow Folly Beach Road to Atlantic Ocean.*

On Highway 301 at the west end of the bridge over the Savannah River, I stopped to read a sign saying that in 1776 Robert Dunne began operating a ferry here. This was a gateway to the west for the settlers from the Carolinas and Virginia.

Shortly after setting foot in South Carolina, I heard shooting a short distance from the road. This set me to worrying that some damn fool could fire in my direction.

Later my fears grew when some hunters stopped to ask for directions to a hunting club. I thought, If they're out here with guns and know nothing about the area, how do they know they're not shooting toward the highway?

Another thought: We will have close to 3200 miles when we finish. How much farther could I go? Physically I could go on, but psychologically I would weaken. I think I'd lose the will to continue quicker than I'd lose the physical ability.

On the basis of a couple of experiences I decided that police officers sure do dress informally around here. Parked for a pit stop, Elaine had one stop to ask her if she was in trouble. He was dressed in an orange T-shirt and shorts.

Later one asked me if I needed help. He wrote Levis, a T-shirt, and a ball cap that said, "Dixie, God's country."

On our second evening in South Carolina, Elaine and I talked about how our daily routine has evolved in a most surprising way. Before leaving home, we'd planned on starting each day's run at about seven o'clock.

At the time I thought that was really early. Yet after two weeks on the road we found ourselves rolling out of bed between 4:00 and 4:30 A.M., and running within an hour by Elaine's headlights or my flashlight.

Our modus operandi has been that I run three miles to where Elaine is parked for a pit stop. I eat and drink what she has prepared, and we visit. Then I shove off for another three miles.

And so it goes until we finish the 26 miles. That has been our routine, which we'll vary only on the last day when I'll run 5.2 miles to time our finish for media coverage.

The problem I ran into with the last few miles was that Highway 278 was the only road leading to the popular Hilton Head Island vacation area. As a result I had to contend with a mess of traffic. It set me to worrying, My God, what a time to get hit with so few miles left!

At one point on my next-to-last day, and last day of long distance, I said to myself, We're getting very close to finishing our 3192 miles. The question is, What have we accomplished? I came up with these answers.

1. A hidden reward of our run, one we had not anticipated, is that it has brought Elaine and me closer together. We both realize this is something we did together. And when it's over, we will share, as equal partners, the satisfaction of accomplishing what we set out to do.

2. For 20 years, ever since reading *My Run Across the USA* by Don Shepherd, the challenge of a transcon run was on my mind. Could I do it? With Elaine's help, I've met that challenge.

3. Elaine and I were able to meet our goals. We met our goal of averaging 26 miles a day (the final figure will be 26.08). On back roads we met people and saw places that increased our knowledge of our country and reawakened us to its diversity, its size and its strength.

4. From the time we started, Elaine was firmly resolved that I would not lose weight. Her nourishment crusade has been successful because I lost only five pounds – less than any other transcon runner has reported.

5. By the grace of God we were lucky in that neither of us had any serious illness nor injury during our 124 days on the road.

6. We believe that our run made the statement about aging that we intended.

7. We remained in action for 124 days, never taking a day off – which is another manifestation that senior citizens have more physical stamina than they are credited with.

After months of struggling out of bed at 4:00 or 4:30 A.M., lounging there on our last day until seven seemed almost sinful. This last day was purely ceremonial, only 5.2 miles and timed to arrive at the ocean at a time set by the media.

The thought that kept running through my head – as it often did during the past few days – is, I can't believe that we really did it.

As I headed for the finish, my spirits were buoyant. It was a beautiful, beautiful world! Especially if I didn't miss the turn at Folly Field Road and mess things up.

Nearing the beach, I spotted Elaine standing beside a walkway. Two men were with her, and she introduced them as newspaper reporters Mike Miller of the (Hilton Head) *Island Packet* and Bill Caton of the *Savannah Morning News*.

They suggested that I run across the beach and into the Atlantic before they conducted their interviews. I tried to get Elaine to run with me, but she balked, saying, "It's your moment."

I didn't feel that way. It was OUR moment. But she was adamant, saying, "I want to camcord the finish."

I struggled across the sand, damn glad that I didn't have to run far in it, and into the Atlantic.

Splash! Water never felt so good!

Elaine followed and dipped her hands in the ocean. "Just wanted to feel it," she said.

Elaine and I were standing on the beach, answering the many questions of Miller and Caton when a TV reporter from Channel 11, a CBS affiliate, showed up. At his request I ran into the ocean again so that he could photograph my finish. As I did so, I thought about my Marine classmate Joe Hall who had arranged all this media coverage.

We chatted with all three reporters for almost an hour before they departed for other assignments. We were impressed with the interest all three showed in our run and the intelligence of their questions.

After reporters left the beach, Elaine and I stood at the ocean's edge with arms around each other, enjoying the water splashing over our feet. We were silent awhile, then I asked, "What are you thinking?"

Without any hesitation, she said, "That it's over – and yet that it will never really be over. It's something that will always be with us, as part of us – just yours and mine."

I nodded an affirmative, then Elaine said, "Now tell me what you're thinking."

"Well, I don't know if I can express it," I answered. "But I've been asking myself how were we able to do it. And I've sort of decided we did it because we controlled our own destiny.

"We lived by what we did – or what we failed to do. We were accountable only to ourselves. No board, no CEO, no president, no general, no boss told us what to do and what not to do.

"We marched to the beat of our own drummer. And also we were able to do it because we were lucky."

Hugging me, Elaine said, "And don't forget God. We both prayed a lot."

"We sure did," I replied, "and God smiled on us."

FLORIDA

Dates: *October 11th to 13th, 1996*
Miles: *46.3*
Route: *Start at Alabama/Florida border on Highway 29 and follow 29 south to Pensacola. Follow Palalox Street to Palalox Park, then Main Street and Bayport Parkway to Pensacola Bay, and south Florida border.*

DAY ONE. Interesting how one thing sometimes leads to another. In September, as Elaine and I were about to leave for a Tauck Tour of Florida resorts, she said, "Too bad you're not running across Florida when we are there for the tour."

She was referring to the fact that Florida was one of the 24 states we had not run across. Presto! With her words into motion went thoughts about running across Florida. They crystallized when we began our Florida run today.

The thinking went like this: We had run all the other states south of North Carolina. When we would begin our state runs in 1997, we would have to dip far south to do Florida. But – and this was the thought that grabbed us – if we could run Florida separately, we could go directly to North Carolina next year and save miles and time by not having to swoop south to Florida.

Studying the Florida map, I saw that it was less than 50 miles across the Florida panhandle in the Pensacola area. I told Elaine we could fly to Pensacola and complete the run leisurely in 2.5 days. She bought the idea.

Florida would be unique in that we'd done all the previous 26 state runs with Elaine pit crewing from our motorhome. In Florida she would be pit crewing from a car, and she was a bit apprehensive about this until I reminded her she had once pit crewed a 166-mile race for Dr. Ralph Paffenbarger and me while driving a car and not a motorhome.

We were both aware that the most convenient feature of the motorhome that would be missing would be the commode. We maneuvered around this by – and pardon the graphics here – bringing a plastic bucket and plastic bags to line it with and to dispose of with each (ah, euphemism here!) voiding. A realistic problem, a practical solution.

Our game plan included such logistical considerations as a small ice chest, first-aid supplies, food (such as small cans of beans and fruit, cookies, Powerbars, candy), and running gear for heat and rain. We bought a large duffel bag that held all this running gear.

So equipped, with Elaine driving a Hertz Mercury Sable rental, we arrived at the Florida/Alabama border on Highway 29. Our route would follow Highway 29 all the way to Pensacola Bay.

On the drive from Pensacola to the start I found myself thinking of some impressions I held of Florida. The freshest was of the Tauck Tour a couple of weeks previous – the luxury of the Marriott Resort on San Marco Island and of the Boca Raton resort; of seeing a dozen alligators; of visiting Cape Canaveral and vivid reminder of the Challenger tragedy in 1986; of visiting Key West and of being surprised by the staggering cost of real estate and by the hordes of homosexuals, and of treading on history when visiting the Truman summer White House.

All my other impressions of Florida were sketchy. From history I knew the state was loyal to England in the Revolution and to the Confederacy in the Civil War; that Miami was a place I had no desire to visit again; that in recent years Florida was home to some great college football teams; that the campus of the University of Florida in Gainesville was quite attractive (I'd spent three days there being examined as a guinea pig in Dr. Michael Pollock's study of older athletes.); that the state was known as the "Sunshine State" (why else would I be running there in October!); that St. Augustine is the oldest continuously occupied community in North America.

At the border I saw that the Alabama/Florida boundary sign was planted atop an overpass over railroad tracks and at the northern edge of the town of Century. A well-defined area compared to the many nondescript state borders where I have started runs. In 30 yards I passed a Piggly Wiggly market and, across the street, some deserted store fronts.

Piggly Wiggly brought on a smile. Back in my grammar school days Piggly Wiggly pioneered self-serve markets in the Sacramento area.

Every so often some of my compatriots and I would descend on the store and confiscate candy or other goodies. Lucky for us there was no surveillance. At the time, we regarded self-serve markets as a passing fancy thinking they'd never withstand raids such as ours.

Even though Century was a sprawled out community (I followed sidewalks through it for over two miles), the only businesses I saw were Piggly Wiggly, a Dollar Store, Bill's Market and a used-car lot. I got the impression, mainly from seeing much substandard housing, this was an impoverished community.

A luxury home on the southern edge of town seemed completely out of place. I had not seen even a middle-class home, yet here was this place with an indoor pool, tennis courts, three-car garage (itself palatial compared to some of the homes), and I'd guess from its size, five bedrooms.

I had gone less than a half-mile when I saw the First Tabernacle Baptist Church, the first of four Baptist churches seen during the day. Yep, I'm in the South.

The most distinctive was Pleasant Hill Baptist Church, about seven miles south of Century, and established in 1856. About it were at least 300 graves in a setting under pine trees. I took time out to check a few graves and found some dating back as far as 1857.

I was comforted by Highway 29 being a divided highway with a grass median in the center because this meant, as I ran facing traffic, I did not have to worry about a car passing from behind hitting me. There were two lanes on each side of the median.

Most of the time I had a 30-inch bike lane. Outside the bike lane was a 10-foot shoulder of grass.

At first Elaine had some qualms about parking on the grass shoulder. She thought the police might ticket her.

It didn't take long for us to realize that parking on the shoulder was perfectly permissible. In California the scenario would be: Seeing her parked on the shoulder, a CHP officer would brake to a stop, whip out his citation book and give her a ticket.

For the most part I was able to run in the bike lane, but there were some miles when I had to run on the grass shoulder. My concern there was snakes.

Early in the day I stopped to ask a construction worker building a new Burger King if there were any snakes in the grassy areas along the road. His answer, "Shouldn't be too bad, I reckon." Wasn't quite sure what that meant.

For her part Elaine reported that each time she was parked for a pit stop she had several offers of help. She was favorably impressed with the friendliness of the Florida folks and pleased that parking on the grass shoulder was permissible. Her one frustration was not being able to sight an alligator in any of the creeks or waterways along the route.

In the rare times today that I would pass by a cleared area, it stood out in stark contrast to the prevailing heavily forested areas that lined both sides of the highway. I saw little evidence of agriculture, just a couple of hay fields and a cotton field – the latter moving me to break into a chorus of "Dixie" which in turn moved the alligators as far away as the Everglades to wail.

Along the day's route there was not too much to be seen, yet some scenes did leave an impression. Like these:

- Just past Century, a shanty where four tots, ages two to four I'd guess, romped unsupervised in a muddy yard filled with debris and a horse lay in the mud nearby. No fence to restrain these kids from wandering onto the highway. Leaving me to wonder, What chance do these little black kids have in life; and, on the flip side, Michael Jordan making $40 million a year. No wonder he can smile.

- Beside the flat road and just out of Century a white cross to memorialize a traffic death. Not only is the road flat, but it is divided and there are no curves. How did this fatality happen?

- When I went by Green's Monuments at six miles, I asked myself, "Why are these mementos of our mortality always so much more poignant or subjective as we grow older? Even as I asked the question, I was aware that the number-one concern of older people is not death but fear of loss of independence. The monuments brought on a chuckle when I recalled a scavenger hunt with Barney Pendergast and Joe Quintana in our high school days. One item on the scavenger list read, "Bring in something very unusual." When Barney, Joe and I showed up at the party with a tombstone monument, people gasped in horror over the thought of our taking a grave marker. It took us a few moments to convince them that we had borrowed the marker from a monument maker.

- At one point today when I saw some kudzu, I was reminded of the first time we ever saw it which was in Georgia. Compared to this stuff, ivy grows at turtle pace. The kudzu we saw in

Georgia had engulfed entire buildings. Which reminded me
that I had better move a bit faster or it would entwine me.
- Beside a deserted home, enclosed by a cyclone fence and
confined within were eight goats, six of them youngsters, bah-ing
their heads off – leading me to believe in a food shortage here.
- Real-estate insight: for sale, 13 acres, custom home, $120,000 firm.
- In the hamlet of McDavid all I saw were Watson's Convenience
Market, a gas station, volunteer fire department, and a few homes.

I had no problem with drivers or traffic today with one exception: In 27 states of running the one invariable has been the aggressive and inconsiderate drivers of oversized motorhomes.

So fed up with them was I at one point today that I did a no-no:
As one approached, I decided to stay on the fog line and see if he
would move over and give me a little running space.

He didn't, not an inch. When he was 30 yards in front of me, I
jumped onto the grass for the sake of mortality.

Conversely, when the truckers become aware (through their CB
chatter) of what I am doing, they generally move over and give me
room. By the time I was halfway through the day's run, word must
have spread to the truckers that an old man was running the road
because most of them did move over for me.

Because I had logged a daily average of only five miles for the
preceding two months, I was at a loss to understand why the day's
run was so easy. I had expected to be tired and dragging. I wasn't.

The only problem I had came at about 13 miles when my groin
and thigh muscles began to act up. I took remedial action by putting
on a pair of compression shorts under my running shorts, and the
result was a return to normal.

The day's run came to an abrupt stop at 21.1 miles because Elaine
announced, "I'm tired, that's it."

She caught me completely by surprise at a time when I was
thinking of going 23 or 24 miles, hoping to cut the run to two days.
A runner does not have to be a rocket scientist to know the com-
mandment, "Honor thy pit crew, for the pit crew is thine life blood."

Meekly I responded, "Okay." Actually I felt good just getting 21.1
miles today and a little guilty at not recognizing that Elaine's pit
crewing is tiring, too.

Our finish was directly across the highway from the Alendale

Methodist Church. Just as we were getting ready to drive back to Pensacola, the minister came out from his residence and asked if we needed help. Not today, we said, but maybe you can pray for another day of nice weather tomorrow.

DAY TWO. Yesterday began on a note of uncertainty because we had some questions: Would the police give Elaine any trouble when she parked on the shoulder for pit stops? How would the pit crewing from a car go? Was the road satisfactory for running?

Since I had such a weak training base, would I be able to log 20 or more miles? Would Florida stay true to its reputation as the "Sunshine State" or would it rain?

Today we knew the scenario: Elaine would have no problem pit crewing, the route was satisfactory for running, I was running better than expected, and the weather prediction was for fair weather. We knew the routine; now it was time for the performance.

As we started in front of the Alendale Methodist Church, I had expected the minister to come out and bless our mission. But that was not to be because he was busily occupied riding a power mower while cutting the grass around the church.

I immediately took note that I was starting on a slight uphill gradient. Much more perceptive than yesterday when I ran a dozen miles before I realized that the road, instead of being flat as I had expected, made its way up and down a series of small hills.

And such was its course today for the first 14 miles, until I came into a built-up area. Never was I worried, though, about coming upon a big hill because I knew the highest elevation in all of Florida is only 345 feet. These first 14 miles, similar to yesterday, the road was bracketed on both sides by heavy forest growth except when it passed through communities.

The two communities I went through today were Molino and Cantonment. Not much to see in Molino – just a convenience store, a gas station, clothing store, cafe and a sprinkling of residences. The main difference between the residences seen today, versus the shanties of yesterday, was that today's were mostly middle-class homes.

The main attraction in Cantonment was a manufacturing plant. From a mile away I could see the smoke pouring out from it. Enough to drive an environmentalist into a St. Vitus dance.

In Cantonment I came across a cheerful-looking black guy and asked him what the plant manufactured. "Paper," he said.

Being told this didn't make me feel very bright because I should have been able to deduce from the experience of having Frank Bacon, a friend and retired Marine colonel, escort Elaine and me through a similar paper factory in Savannah. Frank's family was associated with the enterprise.

Elaine and I had a question about how Cantonment was pronounced. The same black guy gave us the answer: "Can-TONE-ment." Hardly vital information, but it did satisfy our curiosity.

I'm a sucker for historical markers, and when I caught sight of one on the golf course in Cantonment I crossed the road to read it. I learned that Cantonment was the site of an encampment of General Andrew Jackson's troops in 1814 on a punitive expedition against the Spanish in Florida and again when he visited Florida in 1821 when he awaited transfer to Florida as provisional governor. I never knew until now that ol' Andy was a provisional governor of Florida.

The road flattened at 14 miles when I came into the built-up area that would extend all the way to our finish at 20.1 miles. The last two or three miles were along automobile row, called "Car City" in these parts.

Luckily for me road construction was in progress these miles. One lane was blocked off and, no workers this Saturday, it belonged exclusively to me.

Running conditions were much similar to yesterday's except that, surprisingly to me, the traffic was heavier and there was one stretch of five miles with no bike lane. This meant I had to run the grass shoulder.

Running it, I observed that the grass was laced with heavy deposits of sea shells. Best I could figure the purpose of the shells was to make the shoulder firmer or to prevent soil erosion. Probably wrong on both counts.

When we started today, Elaine and I each had a wish. Hers was to see an alligator; mine to see no snakes. I won; she lost.

However, from a quarter-mile away I did see what looked like an alligator. When I got there, indeed it was – but a tire alligator and not a reptile. "Alligator," in this case, was trucker talk for a piece of peeled-off tire on the highway.

Had my usual exposure to dogs today. As I passed a pecan orchard, a Chow trotted to the fence and growled menacingly. With Kilmer, it was the beauty of a tree; with me, the joy of a fence.

At a used-car lot a mongrel barked but did not move, and I noticed then that he was missing a rear leg.

A bit scary when, day dreaming, I found myself 20 yards from a huge black Shepherd. So close I'd have no escape if he wanted a piece of me. Fortunately he preferred to continue reclining and keeping an eye on me.

I had been day-dreaming because my attention was focused on trying to think which one of W.E.B. Griffin's Marine Corps novels had Pensacola Naval Air Station as a setting. I could not get my brain to click on that.

I had a moment of luxury today. I went past a Burger King and detoured to use the rest room, quite an upgrading from the bushes.

I indulged myself by taking time to clean my dark glasses. Then thinking, hell, I might as well go all the way, I treated myself to a cup of coffee. So pampered, and carrying my coffee, I returned to running the grassy shoulder.

Several times today as I moseyed down the road, I asked myself, Why is this so much easier than I had anticipated? The answer was not forthcoming. Maybe if it were, I'd consider patenting it.

Best as I could figure, maybe it was because I was so occupied ogling and observing that I did not even think about running. Or maybe it was because I was fresh and strengthened from not having had any long runs recently. True, I could not turn in a very respectable performance in a race, but I seemed able to plod along endlessly and without undue effort.

Saw a few things today that were reminders of other things:

- A large pecan grove reminded me of the ones we had seen in Louisiana. The size of these trees was impressive as was the symmetry of the orchard layout. Estimating the trees to be 100 feet tall, I was curious about how the pecans are harvested. Too time consuming and hazardous to climb the trees or use a ladder. My guess was the pecans fall to the ground.
- Campaign signs at frequent intervals reminded me of the forth-coming elections. I observed that the big spenders were Jones running for sheriff, Roberston for assessor, another Jones for tax

appraiser, Childers for state senate. Why were there no Dole or Clinton signs (and, yes, I prefer that billing)? Two guys by the name of Jones reminded me of the old Mills Brothers song, "The Jones Boys." There I go dating myself again.

- Even had a moment when the Reese family name jumped to life. I saw, mounted on top of a telephone pole, a car calling attention to a used-car lot. At first glance the name appeared to be Reese. On second reading it turned out to be *Neese*. No wonder the dog on duty barked at me.

About the time I was nearing the finish line the thought occurred to me that, just as yesterday, I had not been off my feet since starting. With motorhome pit crewing I would have sat down every three miles for grub and grog. Another thought: I was delighted that no insects had swarmed about my legs during all the time I spent on the grass.

Elaine continued to be impressed with the friendliness of the Florida folks. When parked on the grass shoulder waiting for me at pit stops, she had more than 10 offers of help today. She also reported that when she was parked at McDonald's she heard enough blaring boom-boxes to remind her of a similar experience in Louisiana.

I did not see much point in going beyond 20 miles today because doing so would leave us with too few miles tomorrow. As was, when we stopped at 20.1 miles, I calculated that we would have not more than six miles tomorrow.

Our finish spot was at the intersection of Highway 29 and Brent Road, directly in front of Christian Academy – a very impressive private school spread over what I judged to be about 12 acres. The buildings, all painted pink, appeared to be new.

I got the impression that academics was serious business here. I also got the impression that sending a child here dented the family budget. Hey, money well spent!

DAY THREE. Nice thought as I came to the start: In only five or six miles Florida would be history; we will have done what we came to do.

The route was easy, just follow Highway 29 to Pensacola Bay. And probably all flat, as best I could tell.

Before starting at the busy intersection of 29 and Brent Road, I took a studied look at Christian Academy. The impression was about the same as yesterday–a well-designed plant that seemed to reek of dollars, even to the six-foot iron fence that surrounded it.

Once underway the first thing I took notice of was that, unlike the previous two days when hordes of cars descended on me, the traffic was scarce and I went almost two miles before seeing anyone. The first person I saw was a guy who came out of the bushes.

I was glad to see he was no bigger than I. He wore a tattered jacket and jeans that appeared dampened with urination. He was wobbly and smoked a cigarette.

Unsure of him I did pick up the pace for a quarter-mile. When I looked back, he was nowhere in sight.

Shortly after starting, I found myself in a somewhat deserted and rundown area for close to a mile before I came into an industrial area. Leaving the industrial area, I passed some small businesses and residences just before making the transition to the very outskirts of downtown Pensacola.

Just before the road began to ascend a small hill, I saw several large homes of vintage but all well maintained. At one time these were the mansions of Pensacola.

I could not help but note the number of social welfare agencies about: a support education training program, a children's service center, community clinics, American Red Cross and the Florida Department of Health and Rehabilitation.

Just as I was midway up the hill, a small boy riding a bicycle approached me from a side street. My chance to see if the natives were friendly.

"How's everything this morning?" the master conversationalist asked.

"Fine." I noticed his eyes focusing on the cassette recorder.

"Nice bike," I continued. "What grade are you in?"

"Fifth." Real gabby kid.

"Bet your favorite sport is basketball."

"No, it's baseball and I play second base."

Cheez, the kid was opening up. More than a half-dozen words all at once.

"Well, tell me your name and we'll see how it sounds on tape." This said because he had not once taken his eyes off the recorder.

"Justin."

I played the tape back for him, and it was obvious from his enjoyment that he'd never heard himself on tape before.

Leaving Justin and cresting the hill, I had to detour around a divider that had a statue in the middle of it. Unfolding immediately and somewhat surprisingly before me was downtown Pensacola. Elaine was parked nearby, and we took time out for picture taking near the statue.

Continuing on the northern fringes of downtown Pensacola, I passed by a First Baptist Church, an immense brick structure, and actually the biggest Baptist church I'd ever seen. Business was so thriving this Sunday morning that some of the congregation had to park at the Knights of Columbus lot across the street. Talk about ecumenical.

Speaking of things churchly, as is my habit Sundays on the road, I had taken time out for church by meditating and reflecting on things spiritual. Today my thoughts went to that tenet of Catholicism known as confession.

Many (maybe too many) years as a practicing Catholic I had accepted confession without questioning it. These days, though, I cannot - or is it *do* not - accept confession.

One of the reasons, probably the main reason, I never questioned confession was that it seeded relief. Tell those sins to a priest, and I had a guarantee from the Catholic Church that they were forgiven. Thus forgiven, I entered into the "state of grace" and was, until I sinned again, on the Heaven Bound Express.

These days as I dwell on confession, I see no need for the middle man - the priest - being between God and me. Fact is, carrying it to the ultimate, I don't even have to tell God what I've done wrong. God knows.

I must, though, be truly sorry for my errant ways and resolve to amend and not repeat them. End of church services.

As I came into the very downtown section of historic Pensacola, I saw a small parkway extending three blocks or so. Down the center of the grassy parkway was a brick sidewalk and around its perimeter trees, about 20 feet in height. The parkway divided the street.

As I meandered along the brick sidewalk, I heard a voice from the sidewalk calling, "Hey." Then "Hey, mister."

I paid no attention until I next heard, "Hey, runner." Looking toward the sidewalk, I saw two black kids, one about 12 and chubby and the other about nine or 10 and rail thin.

I moved toward them, and the bigger one asked, "You got that recorder thing?" Then it dawned: They must have talked with Justin, and now the repercussion.

They wanted to be recorded and to hear themselves. I took time out and went through the motions. Judging from their grins, giggles and laughter, they appeared delighted with the results.

I had not expected what I saw in downtown historic Pensacola. What caught me mainly by surprise were the many buildings with ornamental iron work characteristic of New Orleans. The awnings, metal and wood, that sheltered the sidewalk in front of the stores was another novel feature.

Many of the store displays were attractive, and I saw not a single vacant store. In fact, at one corner an eight-story building was under construction.

Edging out of the historic district and toward the pier, I paused to do some tallying. Florida, to the best of my recollection, was the first state we crossed without every talking with a sheriff's deputy or Highway Patrol officer.

It was also the first state in which I did not run in the rain. The "Sunshine State" was true to its reputation; the temperature reached the low 80s on each of our running days.

I saw no live wildlife and found a total of 41 cents. I had talked with very few people – the construction worker who commented on snakes, the black guy in Cantonment, the Methodist minister, Justin, and the two black kids in downtown Pensacola.

With Florida we have now run across 27 states. Reflecting on this run, it seemed to be over too soon. I actually found myself wishing I had farther to run. And it was so easy (maybe understandable since it totaled only 46.3 miles including the 5.1 today)

I could hardly believe it was over. I could not recall having those two feelings about any other state I had crossed.

Epilogue

All the running and all the writing completed, I thought back on both the running and the writing with a series of questions, a cross-examining, to evaluate any meaning that they held:

• *Did Elaine and I prove that older people are capable of considerably more than is generally believed?*
We would hope that for me, between ages 73 and 80 to cover 7,646 miles on foot while crossing states, and for Elaine, in her 60s to drive a motorhome over 60,000 miles, offered evidence of that.

• *Will younger people learn any lessons from reading or hearing about what we did?*
Seeing what Elaine and I did at our ages might give them a new perspective on old age. Maybe taking a look at us they might come to realize that if they live a proper life style, they can be very active in their senior years, much more so than they previously believed.

• *Will what I've done send any message to people with handicaps?*
To some degree, maybe. Some people who, like me, have had prostate cancer, or asthma, or a bad back (spondylolsis in my case) will not be inclined to surrender to their handicap but will be steadfast in their resolve to do what exercise they can.

• *What are some of the benefits Elaine and I gained?*
The whole experience added zest to our lives. It helped to bond us even closer. It afforded us an opportunity to explore, appreciate, and better understand our vast and beautiful country and its people. And, yes, it reaffirmed out belief in the power of prayer. It should be remembered that Elaine got to take her dogs on some elaborate vacations! Our togetherness was recognized by Sylvan Kaplan, a Marine Corps classmate and prominent psychologist, who called our RUNXUSA experience "a tribute to a marriage."

• *Do I have any regrets?*
Only one, and that is in the handful of states I shortcutted – that is, I ran from one state border to another on a diagonal (such as south to west) instead of crossing the state on full east-west or north-south route, I wish I had run across those states on a full route. This bothers me to the degree that I am considering spending time, over one-week periods of different summers, running the full route (by flying to the state, renting a car, doing daily runs).

• *Do I feel that I did anything phenomenal?*
No way. The only things extraordinary about what I did is that to date I am the only person to have run across all 50 states, and that I did it between the late ages of 73 and 80. Hundreds of people can do what I have done, do it considerably faster, and much better (i.e., run longer routes in some states).

• *If I had to capsulize the whole experience in one word what would it be?*
Gratitude. Why gratitude? Because Elaine and I were able to accomplish what we set out to do. Because we never lost a day because of illness or injury. Because the motorhome never had a breakdown. Because we were physically and financially able to do what we did. Because in 558 days on the road we were never entrapped in any natural disaster, such as a tornado or flood. And certainly because here I was a guy who never expected to reach age 80, and yet I was out on the road and running. How good does it get?

• *What would we do differently?*
Very little. We'd certainly correct the mistake we made on our USA run when we had a motorhome without a generator, which meant that the motorhome was often sweltering for Elaine during the day when I was on the road and for both of us many nights when we did not have an electrical hookup for the air conditioner. And if I could turn back the clock, I'd made sure that Elaine had a dog on the USA trip to keep her company when I was running. Oh, how a man can mellow – can hardly believe I said that!

• *In a sentence or two, what advice do I have for runners?*
Most important of all, work at enjoying your running – and life. A runner who enjoys will endure and stay healthy. Make the most of

life. Live it intensely because it will pass all too fast. As John Lennon told us, "For too many people, life is what happens when they're planning something else." Or as Thoreau said, "The danger is we might go through life without living." Jimmy Buffett put it a different way: "I'd rather die when I'm living than live when I'm dead."

• *If a person planned to run across the USA or all 50 states, and asked for some suggestions, what would I say?*
The cardinal point I'd make is that it would be empty and foolhardy to try it without a pit crew. The endeavor requires a total commitment by the runner and the pit-crew person. Recognize that you can do more than you think you can. Remember that mindset is every bit as important as physical condition. The running itself is the easy part. The hard part is finding running space, avoiding careless and reckless drivers, the discomfort and sometimes the danger of foul weather, and the cumbersome logistics. The best way to go is for the pit-crew person to drive a motorhome. Throughout, the experience will be filled with peaks and valleys; enjoy the peaks, weather the valleys. Never once forget that one of your best weapons is your sense of humor. Exercise it!

• *Apart from the running experiences, apart from the union with Elaine, what major fringe benefit resulted from my adventures?*
I'd say the writing of three books – *Ten Million Steps*, *Go East Old Man*, and *The Old Man and the Road*. Not (and this is heresy to American materialism) that the books resulted in any financial gain because, considering expenses, liabilities outweighed assets.

• *So, if not for the Yankee dollah, why did I write the books?*
Three direct reasons: (1) I wanted to document what Elaine and I had done, to leave no doubt about it; (2) I wanted to leave a memento for my family and Elaine's to better understand us and to have a lasting memory; (3) I hoped to put a new focus on aging. In the words of Arnold Schwarzenegger, commenting on my USA run, he called it "a giant step forward regarding our concepts about aging. It will awaken people in their 60s and 70s to their inherent physical capabilities… and will provide proof positive to younger people that in their sunset years they will be capable of considerably more physically than they previously believed possible." An indirect benefit from writing the books has been the pleasure and privilege of working with Joe

Henderson. He has given unduly of his time, his expertise and his patience. I admire him greatly as an editor but cherish him even more as a friend.

• *Now that I've run all 50 states, what next?*
The first priority is for Elaine and me to pursue an active life style, exercise being a part of it. Her exercise is walking the dogs three miles every day. Mine is trying to run an average of 4.38 miles a day (130 miles a month, 1560 a year). I have come to believe that a minimum of three miles a day of jogging (as apart from demanding cardiovascular running) is required for conditioning. As for adventurous running, I'd like to return to three states and in each run a longer route than the one I've already run there, doing this over three summer "vacations", one state each summer. Long range, I hope to keep running/jogging/shuffling to the day I die. In fact, it goes beyond that because on my first day in heaven I intend to break four minutes for the mile and 2:10 for the marathon. There might be a problem with that, though: to wit, my getting to heaven!

• *Bottom line, was the whole adventure worth all the time, effort, and expense?* Definitely yes. Both Elaine and I are better because of the experience, which has enhanced our lives. Hopefully, seeing what we have done, some people will take action to better themselves, to stay active and to age gracefully. Secondly, in whatever we do we will continue to heed the words of Langston Hughes' poem:

Hold fast to dreams
for if dreams die,
life is a broken-winged bird
that cannot fly.

Hold fast to dreams
for when dreams go,
life is a barren field
frozen with snow.

We have held fast to our dreams. Pray God we will have more and never let them go.